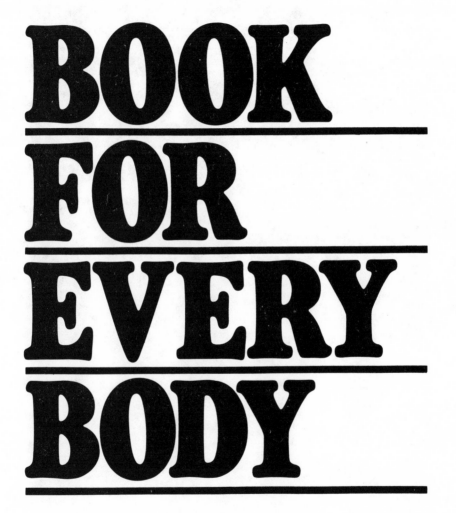

BOOK FOR EVERY BODY

Fitness Exercises for the Entire Family by Benny Crawford

WORLD

World Publications
Mountain View, California

Library of Congress Cataloging in Publication Data

Crawford, Benny, 1946–
    Book for every body.

    1. Exercise.   I. Title.
RA781.C73   613.7'1   78-55792
ISBN 0-89037-132-6

World Publications
Mountain View, California

TABLE OF CONTENTS

INTRODUCTION

The **Book for Every Body** is designed for people who realize that exercise is vital for feeling good, looking your best, and adding years to your life. Without exercise every human body begins to deteriorate more and more each year. The right kind of exercise in the proper amounts will help you offset this deterioration by keeping the muscles in tone, the joints moving freely, and helping the blood circulate efficiently. Without exercise, the body begins to be a detriment to health and happiness and becomes the constant prey of disease and disability.

My purpose in writing this book was not to persuade you to exercise, or to pretend to know the secret to exercise without effort. Exercise is work, and taking care of your body to keep it functioning efficiently, is work—vital work. There is no exercise routine that does not require a certain amount of effort, but the long range rewards are much greater than the effort itself.

The **Book for Every Body** was written to present a concise encyclopedia of exercises including:

- exercises for specific problem areas of the body, including the stomach, buttocks, and waist
- exercises especially designed for men and women
- exercises for pregnant women and post-delivery shape-up
- exercises for off-season athletes
- exercises to get children started in a daily fitness routine
- exercises for couples

These exercises are designed to do the maximum amount of good without the expense of joining a health spa or investing a lot of money in fancy equipment. You can do these sequences anytime and anyplace large enough to swing your arms and legs. They can be done in any comfortable clothing—but loose-fitting clothes are always best for exercise. Wear good shoes with gripping soles on uncovered floors. Bare feet are fine when you exercise on floor mats or on carpeted surfaces.

Once you have made the commitment to exercise, and before actually starting, take a few minutes to review your daily schedule and choose the best time for your session. Some people prefer to exercise first thing in the morning, others before going to bed at night; still others prefer the middle of the day. Whatever your preference, choose a time when you have enough time to warm-up, do the sequences, then cool down, all without rushing. This time should be your own, specifically set aside for exercise and should soon become an ingrained, natural part of your day.

Begin any exercise routine with caution. Do not attempt to "make up for lost time" in one day, or do many repetitions of a specific exercise. Repetitions must be built up slowly for the maximum benefit.

These exercises are designed to put you in shape and keep you in shape for years to come. All you have to do is invest twenty or thirty minutes of your time each day—not a great investment for the rewards of a more efficient and better looking body. But you have to be faithful and sincere about exercising. Routines must be done five days per week, and the two rest days interspersed.

Explore the sequences listed through the book, and start your fitness routine today. The benefits will soon become obvious.

PART 1

FUN EXERCISES FOR THE ENTIRE FAMILY

CHAPTER 1

Awareness: The First Step

Health is no gift—it has to be earned, or at least worked for. Anyone can notice the extreme difference between a healthy person and a sickly person. Barring extreme unforeseen circumstances, we can determine the type of person we will become if heredity gives us the chance.

Our bodies are like machines. If a machine is not properly used and maintained, it becomes stiff, deteriorates, and runs haltingly, if at all. It also wears out much sooner than intended. If it doesn't get the proper type and amount of fuel, it will really degenerate quickly.

The body's fuel is, of course, food. Food is fuel and fuel is burned and must be replaced constantly. Nutritionists have devised an eating plan that provides the body with the essential nutrients. These nutrients are proteins, fats, carbohydrates, vitamins, and minerals. The requirements are called the recommended dietary allowance (RDA), and they can be met by eating from the Four Basic Food Groups, in the specified amounts.

- Meat Group (includes fish and poultry)—five ounces per day
- Fruit and Vegetable Group—four servings per day
- Bread and Cereal Group—four servings per day
- Milk, Egg and Cheese Group—two servings per day

The nutrients essential for the adult RDA are widely distributed in the foods we eat—they cannot be found in any one food item. The proper balance of food is essential to health and longevity.

You may want to shed a few pounds in addition to toning and firming your body by doing the exercises. The safest and best way to accomplish this is to establish a transitional eating habit over a long period of time. The important thing to remember when starting this transitional eating habit is to know how many pounds you want to lose, then give yourself several months to make the change. Once you set your goal, you can start the transition. Begin by identifying the fatty foods you eat, then eliminate one of them for the next two weeks. After you are successful with this elimination, eliminate another one for the next two weeks. Continue this process until you have reached the desired weight. By this time you should have established good, balanced and sensible eating habits.

The important thing to remember when dieting is to concentrate on eating the right foods (RDA) and still getting fewer calories than previously consumed. Exercise is very important when dieting—to tone and tighten muscles. Starvation diets are not a good way to lose weight—they often cause you to lose much more than a few unwanted pounds.

Bodies with chronic functional problems and little resistance to disease and fatigue are often the product of an unbalanced diet. Malnutrition is not just lack of food—it is most often lack of the proper foods.

In the most literal sense, we are what we eat. An ordinary human body can continue to function and even look presentable for a long time, often with extreme abuse and neglect. But this cannot, and does not, last. Health is not inexhaustible—beyond a certain point it must be worked for and carefully guarded. The sooner you realize the importance of maintaining and bettering your health, the better you will look, feel, and live.

It does not take much time to get a little exercise and stay on an adequate, balanced diet. Awareness of the *value* of exercise and proper nutrition is as valuable as doing the right exercises. Awareness is, indeed, the first step to fitness.

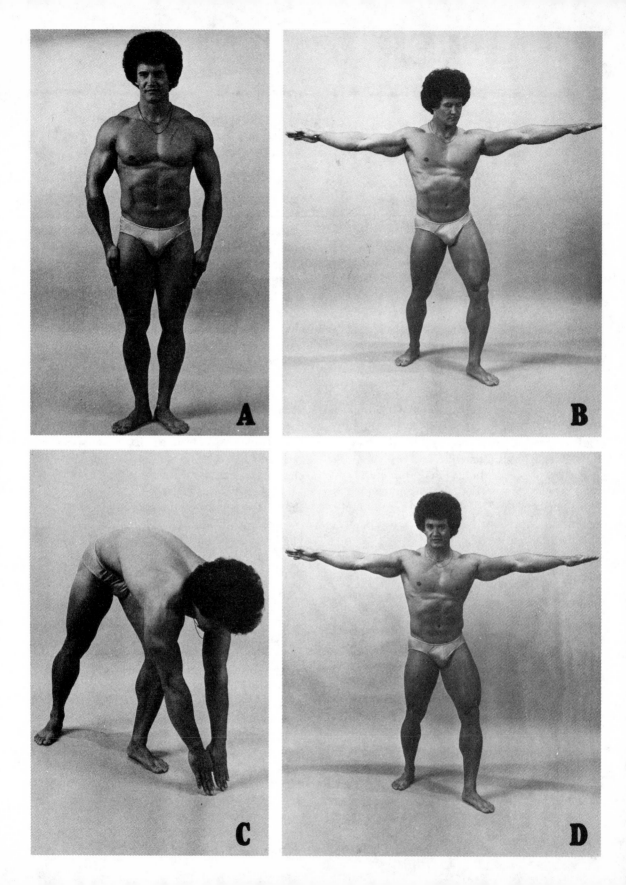

CHAPTER 2

Men's Daily Dozen

The Bird

A *Starting Position.* Stand up straight with your hands at your sides, feet together.

B Step diagonally to the left about one or two feet and simultaneously bring your arms up and out, parallel with your shoulders, palms down.

C Bend at the waist, bring your arms together, and touch the floor two to four inches in front of your left toe, hands together.

D Come back up to the arms out position.

E Pull your leg and arms back simultaneously to the starting position. Repeat exercise with other leg.

Repetitions: 8 (work up to 15).

Benefits: good all around warm-up exercise and body conditioner.

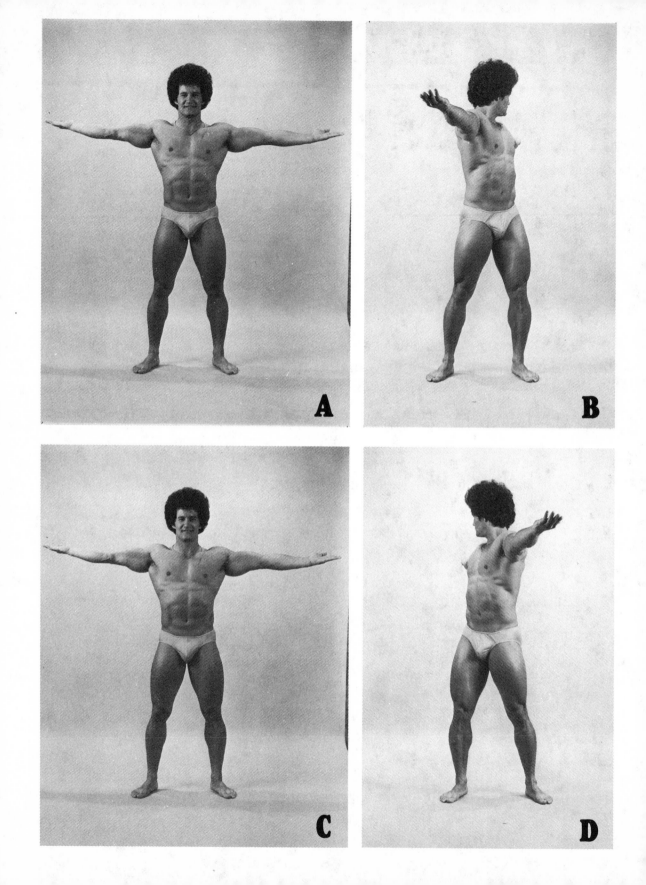

Maytag

A *Starting Position.* Stand with legs spread to shoulder width and arms outstretched, palms up.

B Twist your torso to the left in three short, distinct jerks, until you are twisted around as far as you can go.

C Return back to the starting position after the third jerk.

D Repeat the exercise to the other side.

Repetitions: 8 (work up to 20).

Benefits: shoulder and waist muscles.

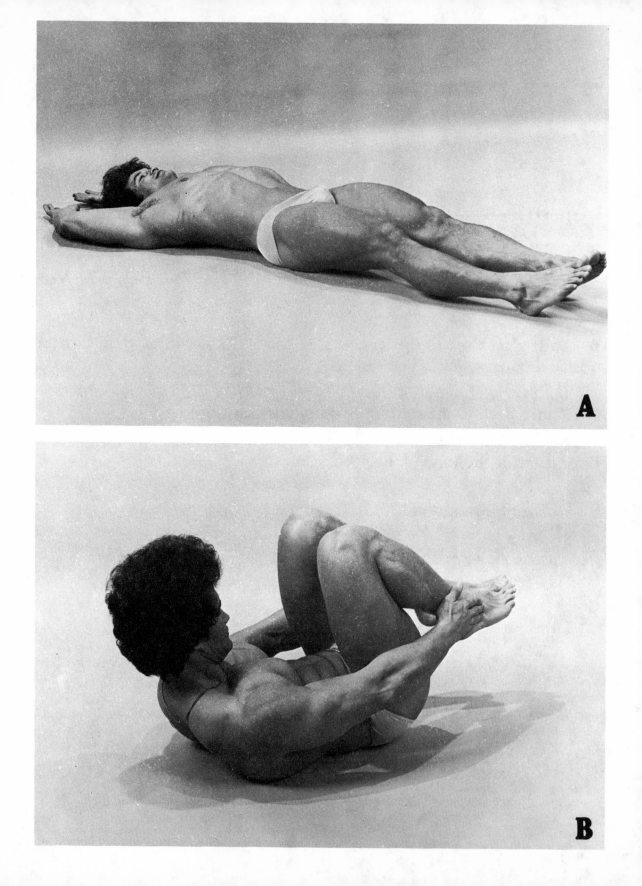

A

B

Ankle Slapper

A *Starting Position.* Lie on your back, feet together, arms stretched out up over your head.

B Taking your weight on your buttocks raise your legs and pull your knees toward your chest (knees bent) and swing your arms around, so your hands can touch your ankles.

C Return to the starting position.

Repetitions: 10 (work up to 40).

Benefits: abdominal and shoulder muscles, and overall condition.

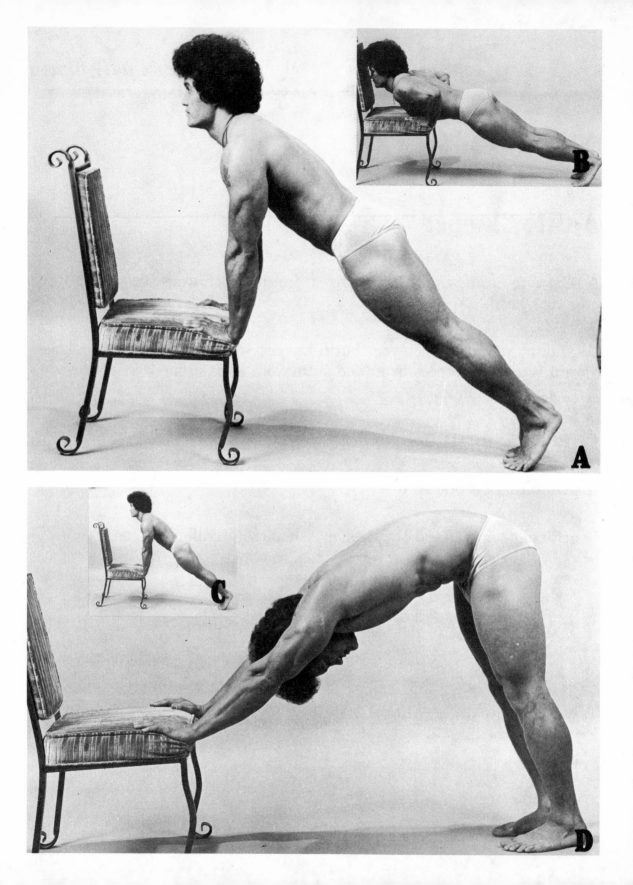

Cantilever

A *Starting Position.* Lean on the seat of a sturdy chair at a forty-five degree angle to the floor, body straight, weight supported on hands and toes.

B Lower your body by bending your elbows, until your chest rests on the chair.

C Push yourself back up to the starting position using your chest muscles. Do two push-ups in this position.

D Now push yourself back at the same time, bring your buttocks up, legs straight, and tuck your head between your arms.

E Bring yourself back to the starting position. Repeat (d) twice.

Repetitions: 8 (work up to 20).

Benefits: chest muscles, back of the legs, shoulder and back muscles.

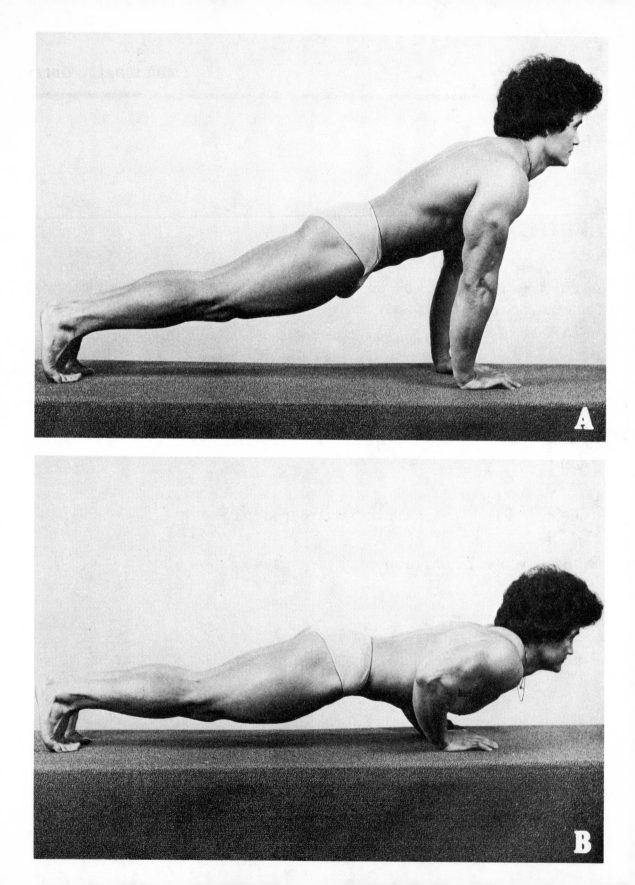

Staple Gun

A *Starting Position.* Do several push-ups but with your hands about two inches apart. As you do them, keep your elbows as close to your body as you can, head up.

B Lower yourself by bending at the elbows and using the triceps muscles to do the work.

C Using the triceps muscle, push back to starting position.

Repetitions: 6 (work up to 15).

Benefits: triceps, chest, and shoulder muscles.

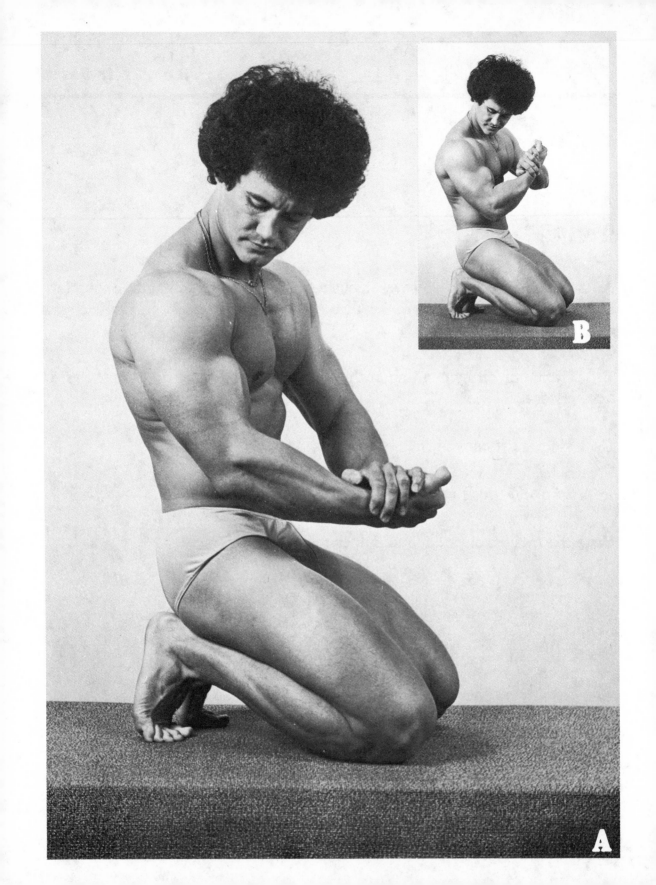

A

B

Cosmic Curl

A *Starting Position.* While in a standing or kneeling position reach down and grab your right wrist (palm up) with your left hand.

B As you push down strongly with your left, bend your right arm upward into a curl.

C Reverse by pushing down with your left, and resisting with the right.

Repetitions: 10 each arm (work up to 30).

Benefits: biceps, triceps, and forearm muscles.

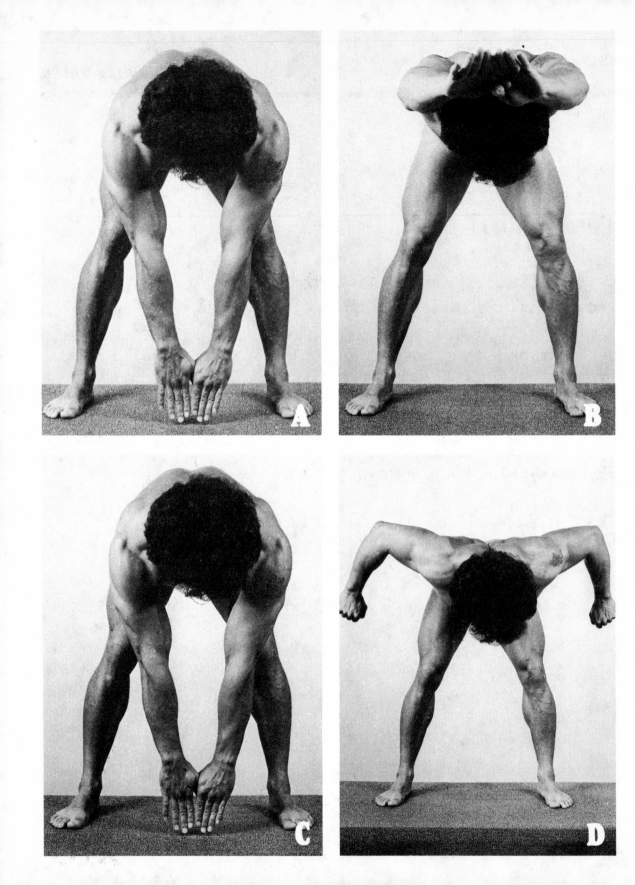

Frog Prince

A *Starting Position.* Get into a "football-hiking" position—legs spread, trunk bent forward, arms hanging down between your legs, thumbs locked with fingers extended, and head up.

B Bring your arms forward and up, and tuck your head down.

C Bring your head and arms back to the starting position.

D Now, unlock your thumbs, and bring your elbows strongly back and up as far as possible. You should feel a strong bunching between your shoulder blades.

E Return to the starting position.

Repetitions: 8 (work up to 20).

Benefits: legs, back, shoulder, arms, stomach, and respiratory system.

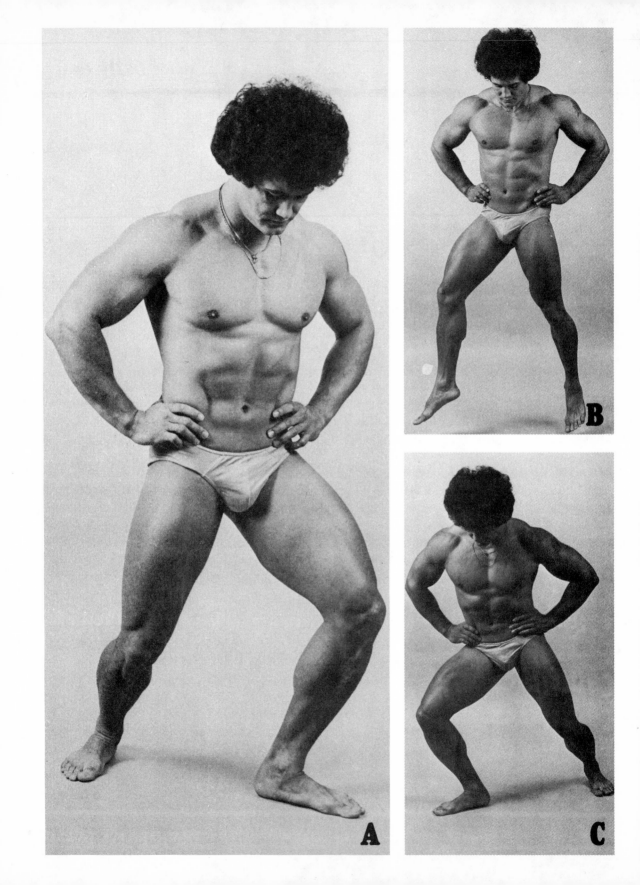

Pogo Stick

A *Starting Position.* Stand with your legs spread, left foot pointed out at a forty-five degree angle and the right foot pointed out to the front. Bend your knees as though you were attempting a squat position.

B Spring up off the floor about a foot, and land with your feet in the reverse position.

C As you land, let your knees bend down as far as possible then spring up and land with your feet in the reverse position again.

Repetitions: 15 (work up to 50).

Benefits: leg muscles, and respiratory system.

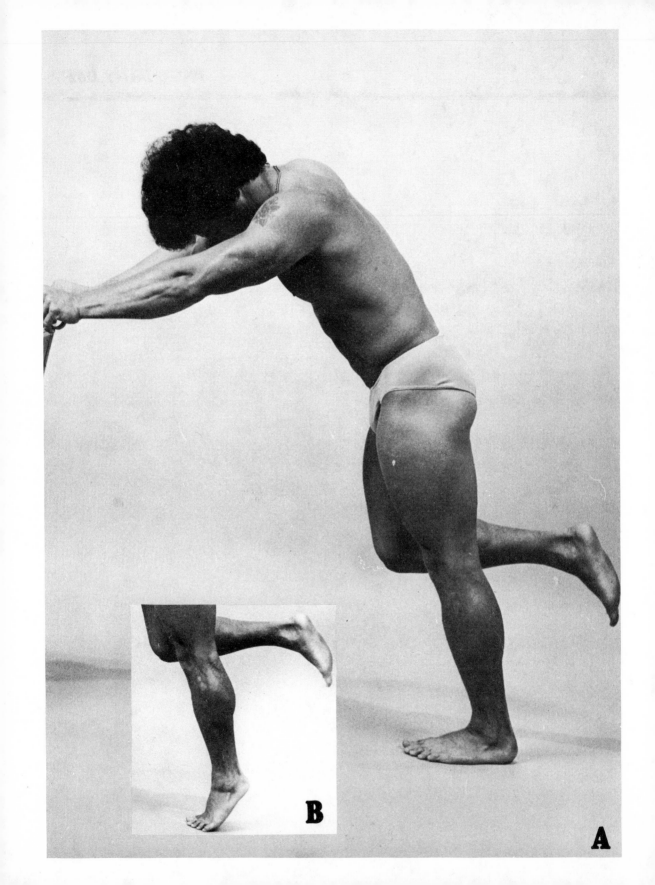

B

A

Lean-To

A *Starting Position.* Lean on the back of a chair with your body weight on your hands and toes. Your body should be in a forty-five degree angle.

B Lift your right foot off the floor and then raise and lower yourself on your left foot using your calf muscle.

C Repeat (b) with the other foot.

Repetitions: 10 (work up to 40).

Benefits: calf muscles.

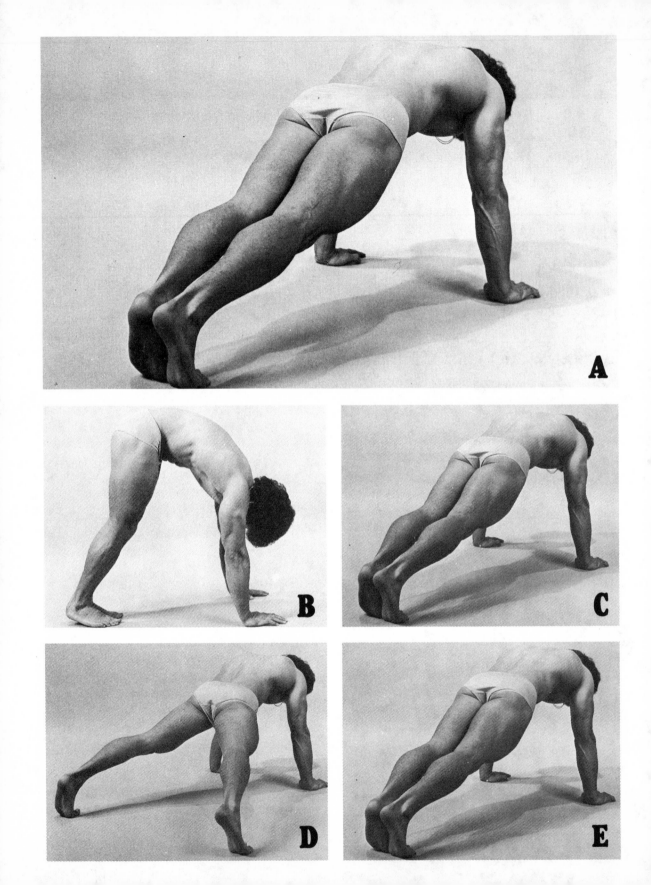

The Obi-Wan Kenobi Hop

A *Starting Position.* Assume a push-up position, knees straight, feet together.

B Trying to keep your knees locked, hop forward so that your feet land as close to your hands as possible, head tucked in between your arms, your buttocks high.

C Hop back to the starting position using your calf muscles.

D With a second hopping motion, spread your legs as far apart as possible, your head and arms remaining stationary.

E Hop back to the regular starting position.

Repetitions: 6 (work up to 20).

Benefits: upper and lower body muscle groups.

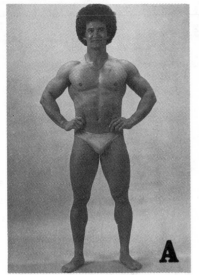

A

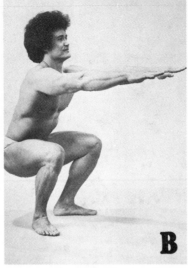

B

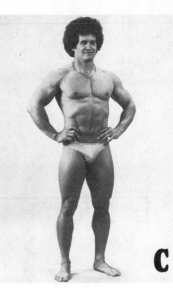

C

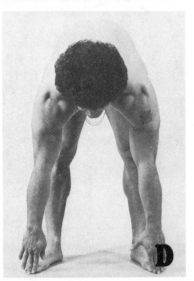

D

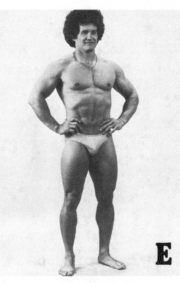

E

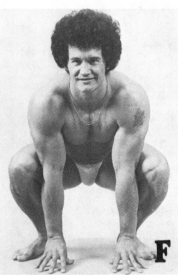

F

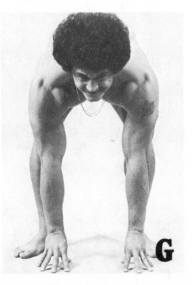

G

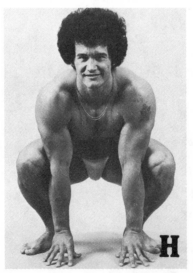

H

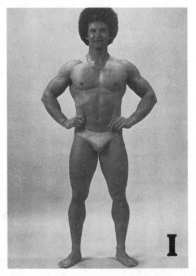

I

Two-Minute Warning

A *Starting Position.* Stand with your legs spread to shoulder width, hands on hips and feet flat.

B Do a deep squat and bring your arms forward and up before you, parallel with the floor.

C Using your leg muscles, push yourself back to the starting position.

D Bend forward at the waist, try to keep knees locked, and touch your toes, keeping head up.

E Return to the starting position.

F Squat again, bending your knees out as far as possible, and bring your arms down between your knees, so that your palms or fingers are on the floor, head up.

G With your hands on the floor, lift your buttocks as high as possible. Your knees should be straight.

H Return to the squatting position.

I Using your leg muscles, push yourself back to the starting position.

Repetitions: 6 (work up to 15).

Benefits: leg muscles and respiratory system.

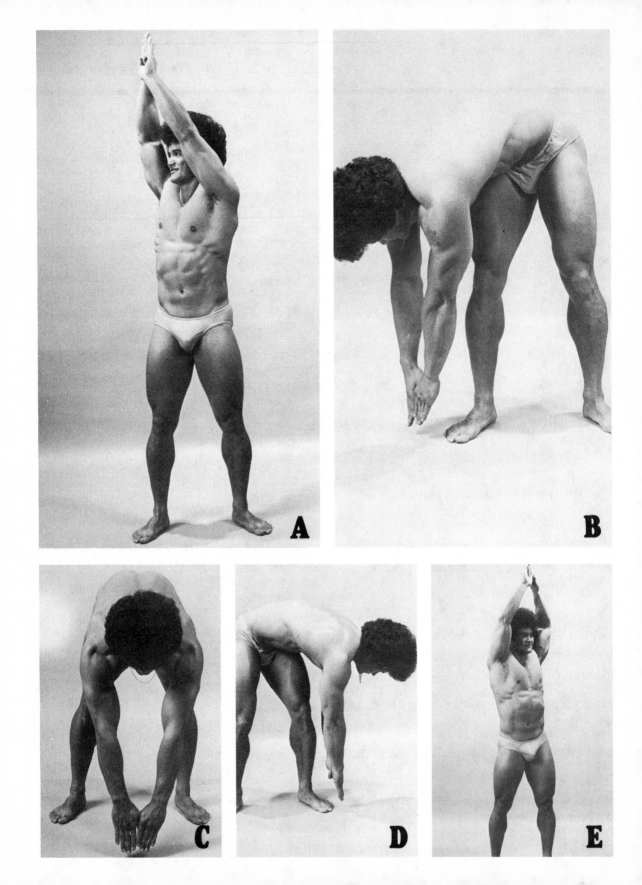

Touching Bases

A *Starting Position.* Stand with your legs spread to shoulder width, knees locked and your hands over your head with thumbs hooked together.

B Rotate your body to the right and bend at the waist so that your fingers touch the floor on the outside of your right foot. Try to keep knees locked.

C Then rotate your body to the left and touch the floor between your toes in front of you, knees locked.

D Rotate further to the left and touch the floor on the outside of your left foot, knees locked.

E Then swing your arms up to the left and back over your head to the starting position.

Repetitions: 8 (work up to 20).

Benefits: back muscles and overall condition.

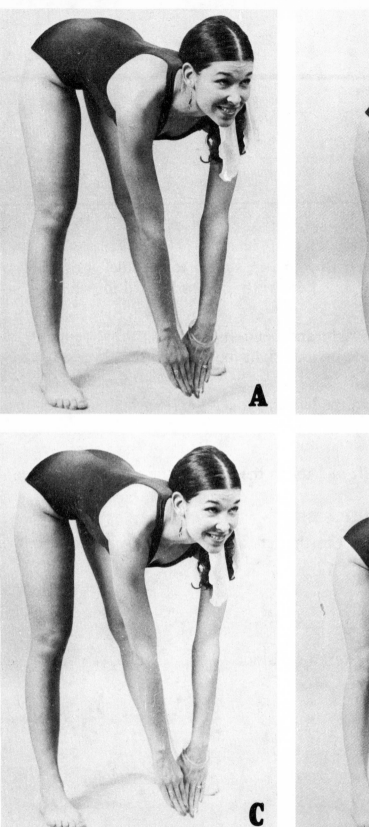
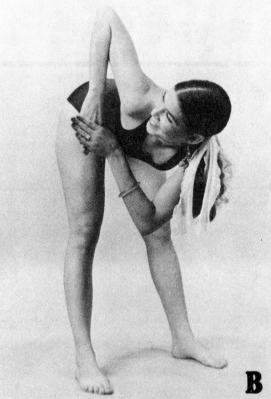
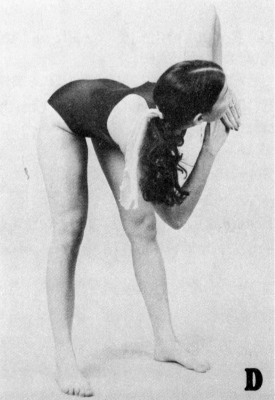

CHAPTER 3

Women's Daily Dozen

The Elephant

A *Starting Position.* Stand with your legs widely spread, your knees slightly bent, and then bend forward from the waist so your fingers touch the floor. Lock the thumbs together. Keep your back parallel to the floor, not arched, and your head up. Your arms, shoulders, and head are the only parts you're going to move in this exercise.

B Twist your bent-forward half to the right. As you do so, pull your right elbow up strongly, drawing your hands against your chest. Pull and twist as far and as hard as possible, looking at your elbow as you do so.

C Return to the starting position.

D Now do the same movement twisting to the left.

E Return to the starting position.

Repetitions: 10 (work up to 30).

Benefits: back muscles, also a good warm-up exercise.

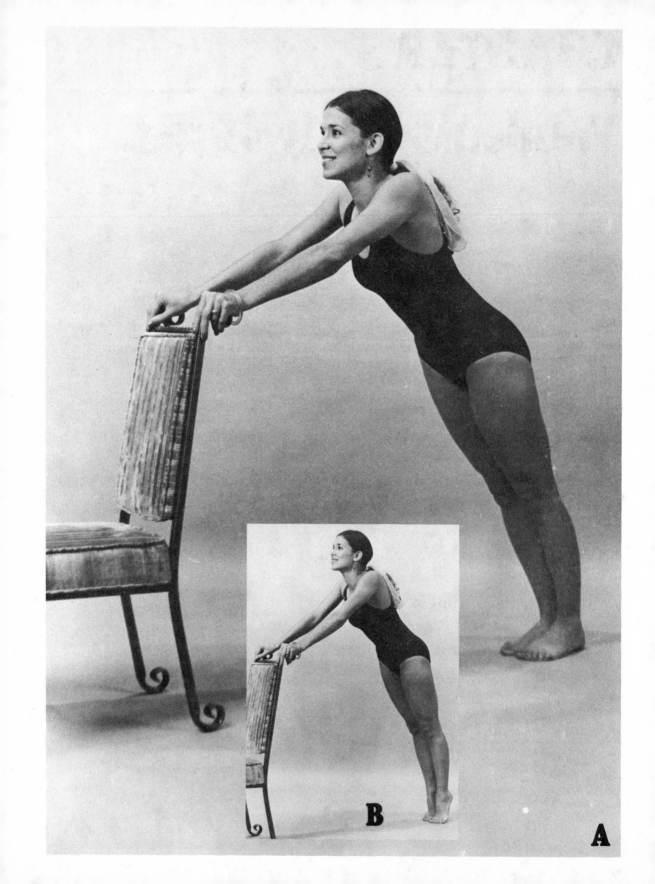

A

B

Flying Buttress

A *Starting Position.* Position a chair so it will not slip. Lean forward with your hands on the chair and your feet flat on the floor. Your body should be at about a forty-five degree angle to the floor.

B Raise yourself up using your calf muscle, get a full extension.

C Lower yourself back again using your calf muscle.

Repetitions: 10 (work up to 60).

Benefits: calf muscles.

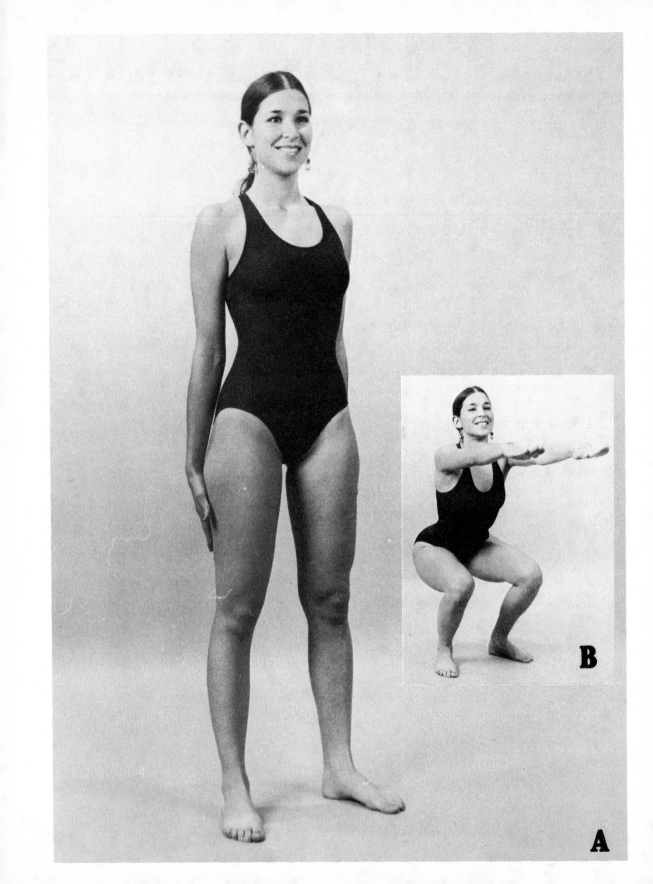

Butter Churn

A *Starting Position.* Stand with your legs spread shoulder width apart, your arms straight down and slightly back, so that your hands are behind your buttocks with the fingers extended.

B Lower yourself into a squatting position, and at the same time swing your arms forward and upward to shoulder level.

C Push yourself back up into the starting position using your leg muscles, while bringing your arms back.

Repetitions: 10 (work up to 30).

Benefits: the upper thighs, and arm muscles.

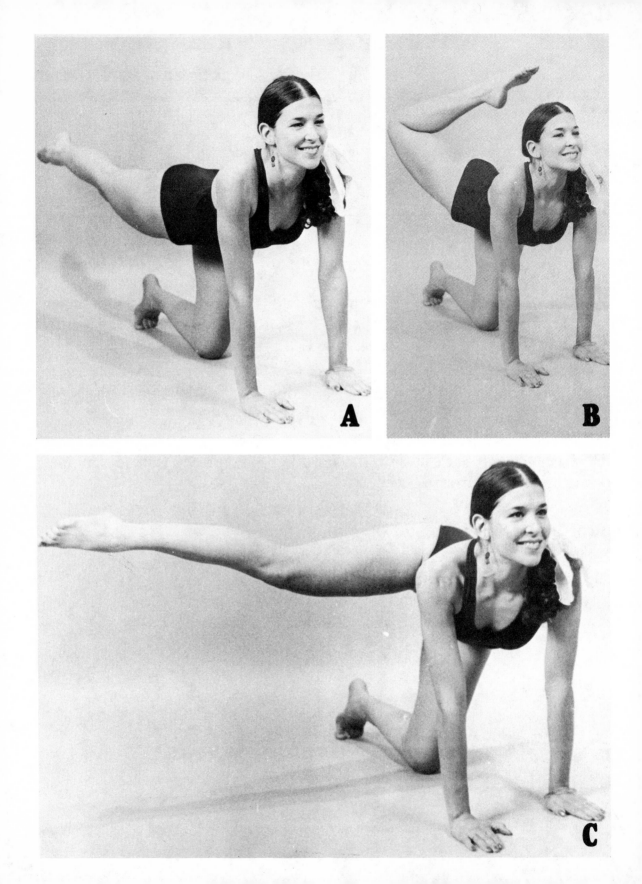

The Tarantula

A *Starting Position.* Get down on your hands and knees, shove your right leg straight back as far as possible, locking your knee with your extended leg parallel to the floor.

B Keep your extended knee stationary, and curl your leg up toward your buttocks. Then straighten and return curled leg to the starting position.

C Rotate your leg outward, extending it to as close to a ninety degree angle to your body as possible.

D Return the leg to the starting position.

Repetitions: 6 (work up to 20 each leg).

Benefits: hip and waist area, leg biceps (back of leg), and lower back.

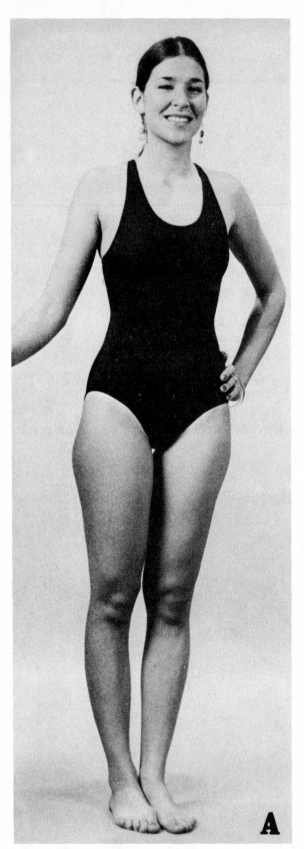

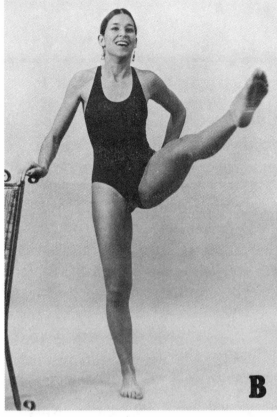

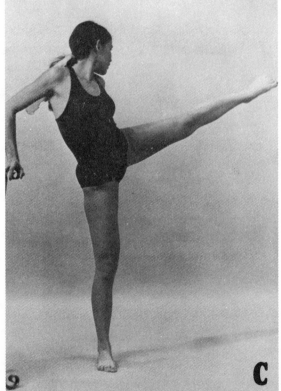

Rocket

A *Starting Position.* Stand with one hand on the back of a sturdy chair.

B Starting with your outside leg, lock your knee, and kick forward as high as you can.

C Return to the starting position.

D Kick to the side and back as far as possible.

E Return to the starting position.

Repetitions: 10 (work up to 20 each leg).

Benefits: leg, stomach and buttocks muscles.

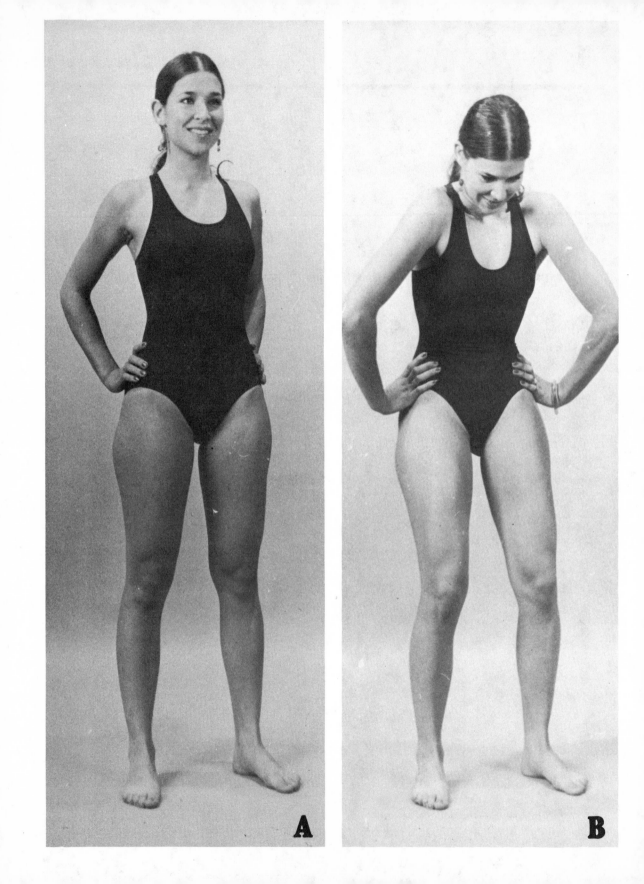

A

B

Wing Flap

A *Starting Position.* Stand with your legs slightly spread, hands on waist, your elbows pulled back as far as possible. (You should feel strong bunching between your shoulder blades.) Keep your head up and slightly back.

B Bring your elbows strongly forward, at the same time hunching your shoulders and dropping your head forward. Hold for a few seconds. (You should feel bunching in your stomach.)

C Return to the starting position.

Repetitions: 10 (work up to 20).

Benefits: chest, shoulders, back, and stomach muscles.

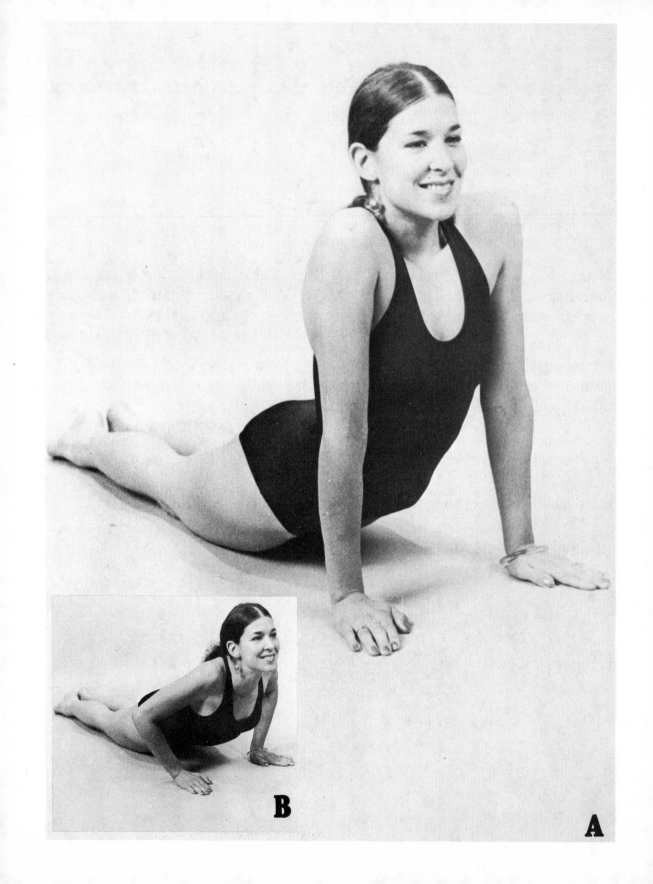

B

A

The Lizard

A *Starting Position.* Lie on floor, face down, legs together, with your upper half supported by your arms. Elbows should be locked, palms to the front, arms a comfortable distance apart.

B Bend your elbows slightly outward, and lower your torso halfway to the floor.

C Push yourself back up using your chest muscles.

Repetitions: 10 (work up to 20).

Benefits: chest, shoulder, and back of arm muscles.

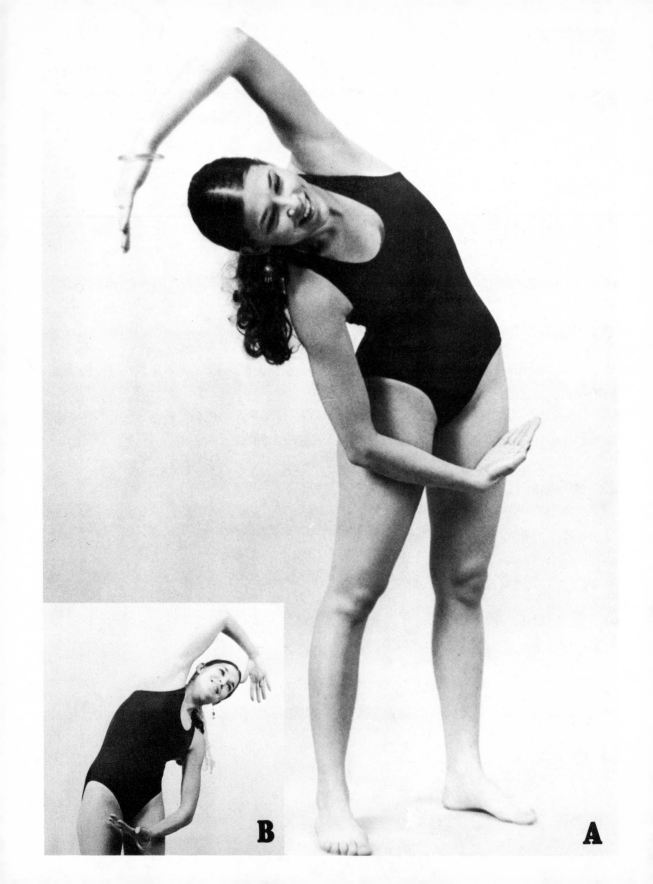

B

A

The Windmill

A *Starting Position.* Stand with your legs spread to shoulder width, one arm up over your head, palm down, slightly bent at the elbow. The other arm should be down in front of you, palm up, also with a slight bend at the elbow, as though you were grasping the rim of a big Hula-Hoop.

B With a wide swing, reverse the position of the arms, bending to the side from the waist and stretch the muscles on one side and bunch them up on the other.

C Reverse the motion to the other side.

Repetitions: 10 (work up to 20).

Benefits: waist and upper back area.

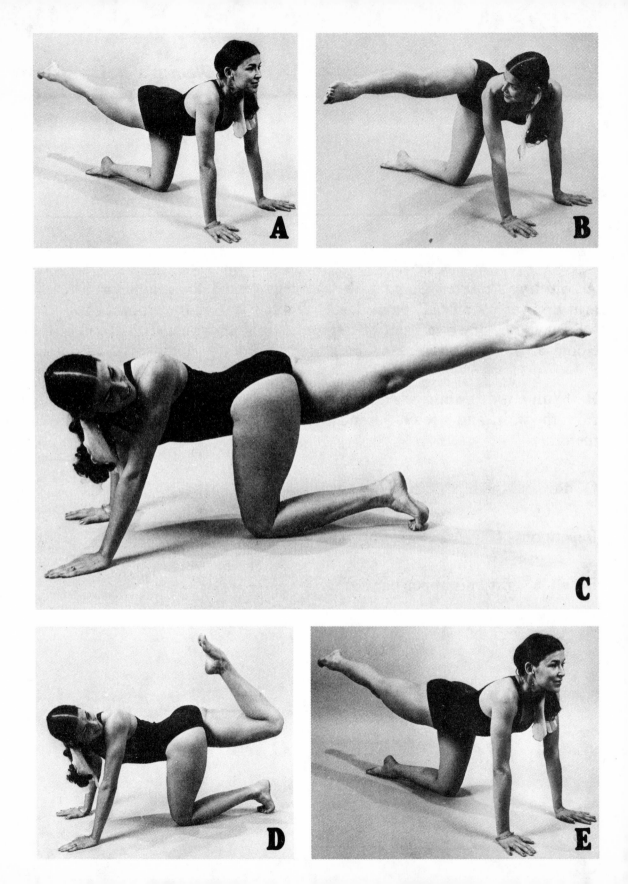

Scorpion

A *Starting Position.* Get on your hands and knees and extend your right leg back parallel to the floor, knee locked.

B Rotate your leg outward, extending it as close to a ninety degree angle to your body as you can manage, turning your head simultaneously to the right looking at your foot.

C Swing your leg to the left simultaneously turning your head to the left looking at your foot.

D At this point curl your leg up toward your buttocks.

E Return to starting position. Then swing your leg back to the right again.

Repetitions: 10 (work up to 20 each leg).

Benefits: hip, waist, buttocks, and leg biceps.

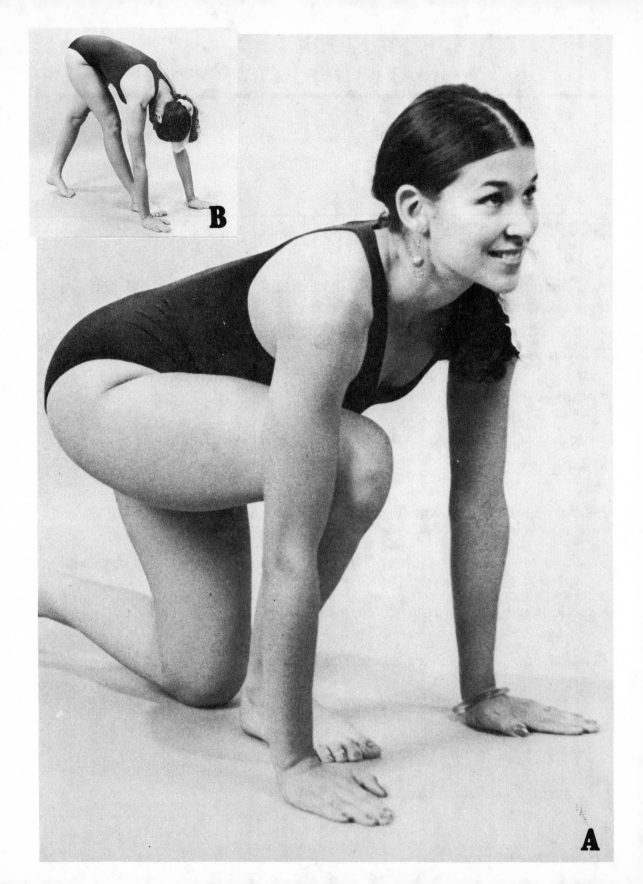

Spring Lunger

A *Starting Position.* Get down on one knee with your arms hanging down, hands touching the floor. The knee on the floor should be in line with the heel of the other foot. Look straight ahead, with your head up.

B Tuck your chin in and simultaneously raise your buttocks up so that both legs are straight, knees locked.

C Bring yourself back to the starting position.

Repetitions: 10 (work up to 20 each leg).

Benefits: neck muscles, back of leg, and buttocks.

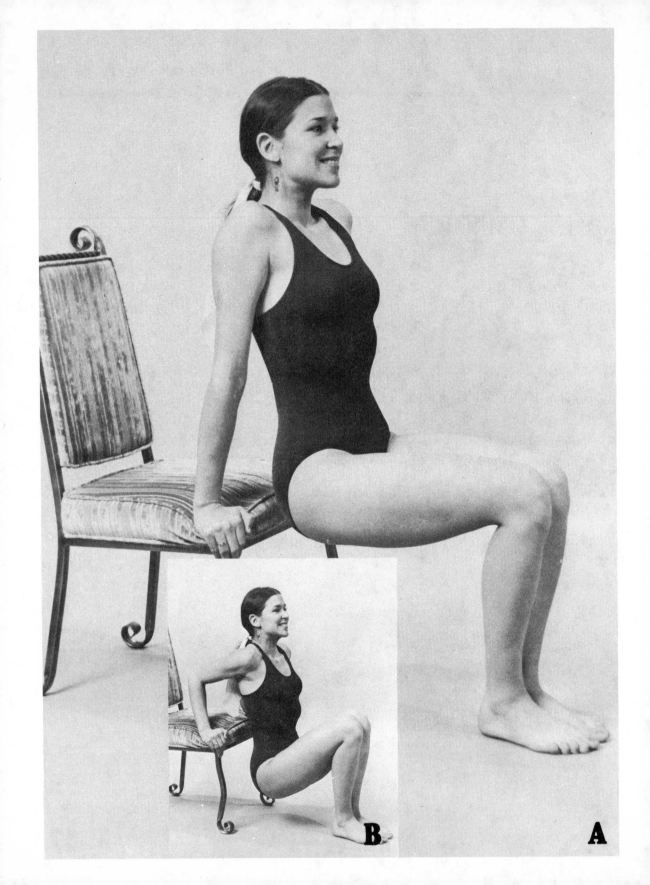

B

A

Backward Pump

A *Starting Position.* Place a sturdy chair against the wall. Squat in front of it with the palms of your hands supporting your weight on the very front of the chair.

B Lower your buttocks as far as possible toward the floor, using the muscles in the back of your arms.

C Push yourself back up using the same muscles.

Repetitions: 10 (work up to 20).

Benefits: shoulder muscles and back of the arms.

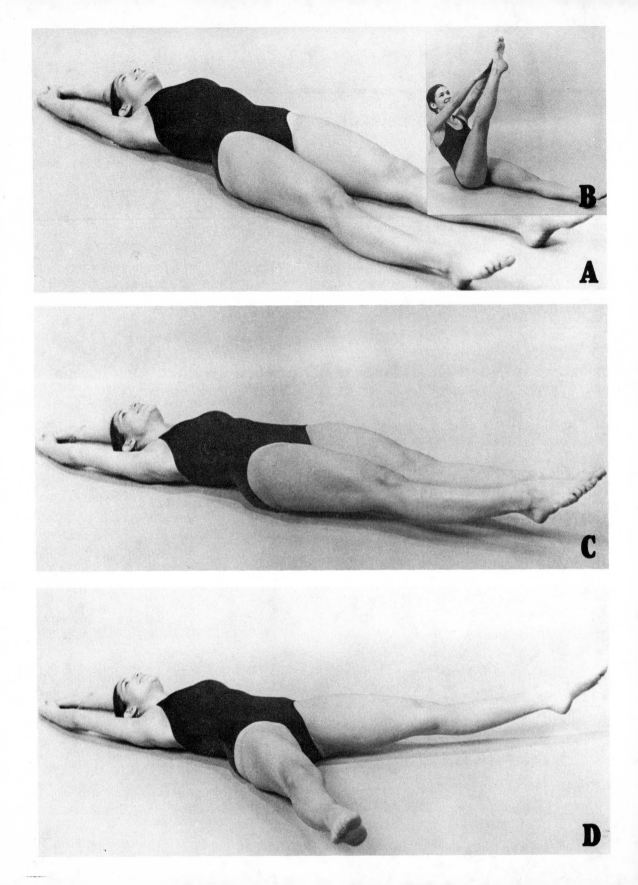

Double Scissors

A *Starting Position.* Lie on your back on the floor with your legs extended and slightly spread, your arms straight out over your head.

B Raise one leg (knee locked) and your arms (elbows locked) simultaneously, and bring them together so that your hands touch your ankle.

C Return to the starting position, and repeat with the other leg.

D Raise both legs (knees locked) two to four inches off the floor and spread them out as far as possible. Bring both legs back to a leg close position. Keep feet off the floor. Repeat.

Repetitions: 4 (work up to 12).

Benefits: leg and mid-section muscles.

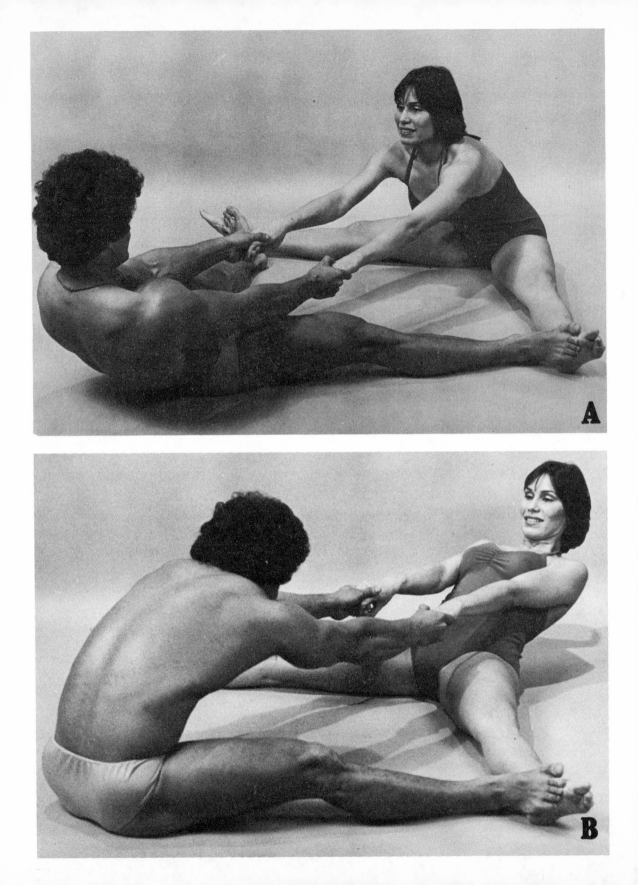

A

B

CHAPTER 4

Exercises for Couples

Locomotive

A *Starting Position.* Sit on the floor facing each other. Spread legs and put the soles of your feet against your partner's feet. Clasp hands.

B See-saw back and forth, one, two. . . . Use your lower back muscles, one to pull, the other to resist.

Repetitions: 15 (work up to 30).

Benefits: lower back, inner thigh, and chest muscles.

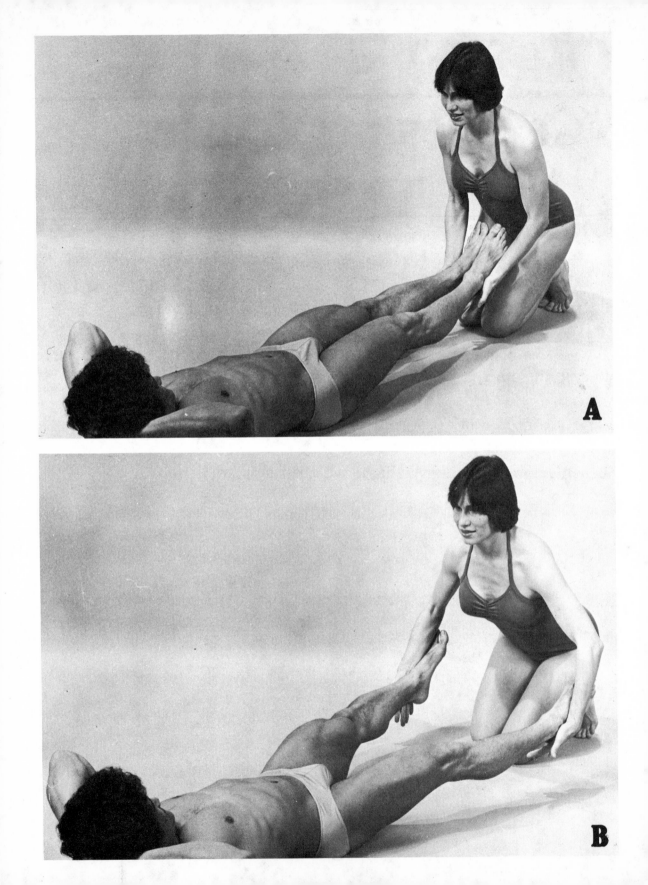

A

B

Hedge Clippers

A *Starting Position.* Lie on your back on the floor, hands clasped behind head, fingers interlocked, head up. Partner should kneel facing you and hold your feet at the ankles with open hands.

B As you open your legs, your partner pushes against the motion.

C To close your legs, your partner pushes them together and you resist. Keep your legs off the floor.

Repetitions: 10 (work up to 25).

Benefits: legs and stomach muscles and your partner's arm and chest muscles.

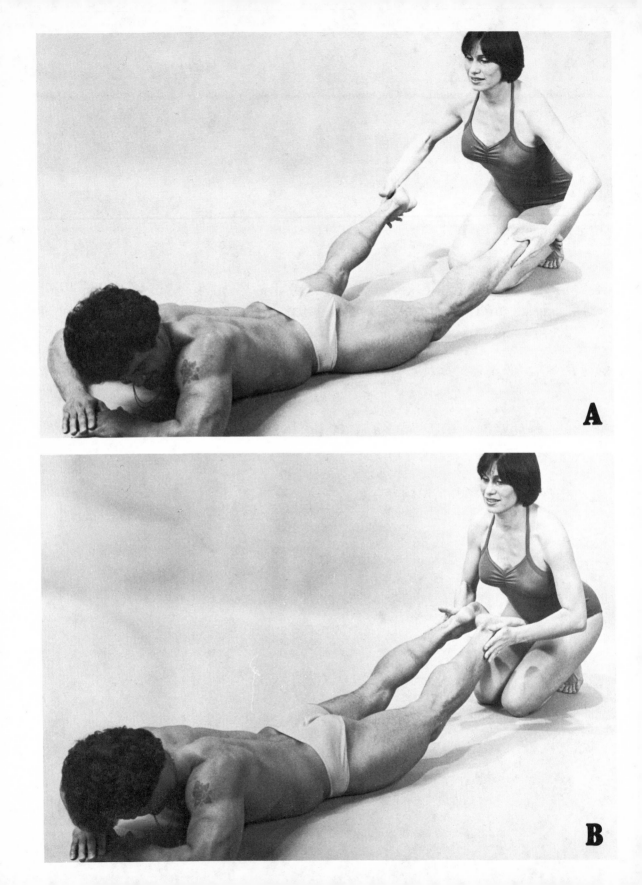

Reverse Hedge Clippers

A *Starting Position.* Lie on your stomach on the floor, one hand on top of the other, head up to keep pressure off the lower back. Partner should kneel facing you and hold your feet on the outside of the ankle, fingers extended.

B As you open your legs, your partner pushes against the motion.

C To close your legs, your partner pushes them together and you resist. Keep your legs off the floor.

Repetitions: 10 (work up to 25).

Benefits: buttocks and leg muscles, and partner's arm and chest muscles.

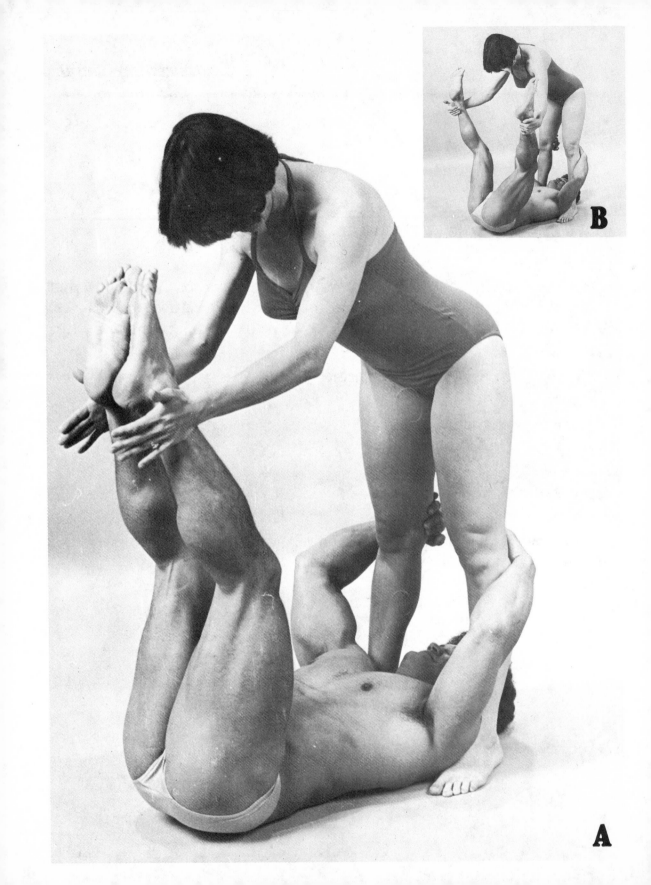

B

A

Cable Cutters

A *Starting Position.* Lie on your back with your legs straight up in the air and your head between your partner's ankles. Reach up and grasp her legs at a comfortable angle. Partner bends forward and grasps your ankles.

B As you spread your legs, your partner resists.

C Your partner pushes your legs together and you resist.

Repetitions: 15 (work up to 25).

Benefits: buttocks, leg and stomach muscles, and partner's chest, arms, and back muscles.

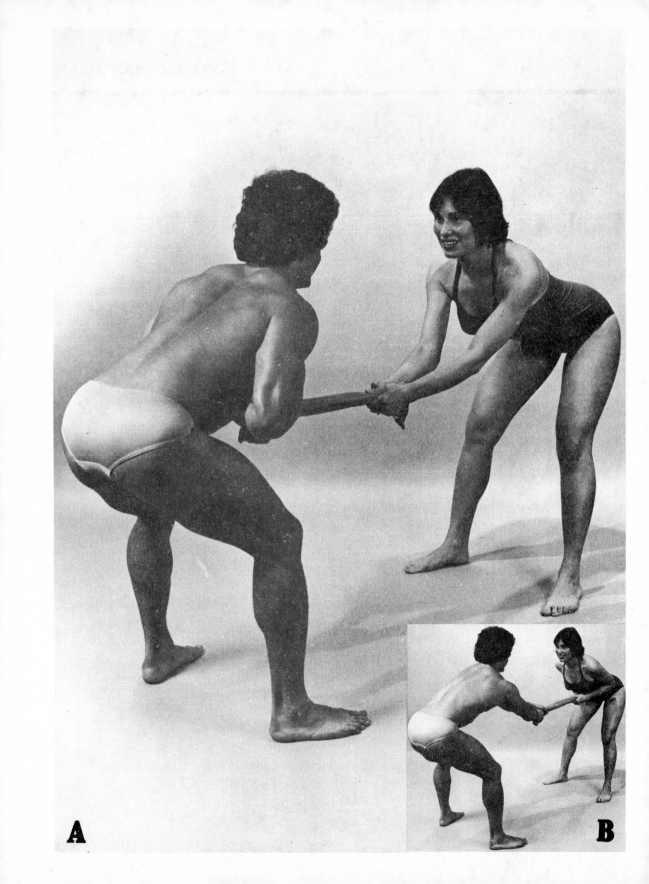

A

B

Tug-of-War

A *Starting Position.* Stand facing each other, bending forward at the waist, knees slightly bent, each holding one end of a hand towel. There should be about two feet between your hands. Your elbows drawn back, and your partner's arms are straight out.

B Your partner pulls and you resist as you extend your arms out. Pull the towel back and forth.

Repetitions: 10 (work up to 30).

Benefits: upper back and arms.

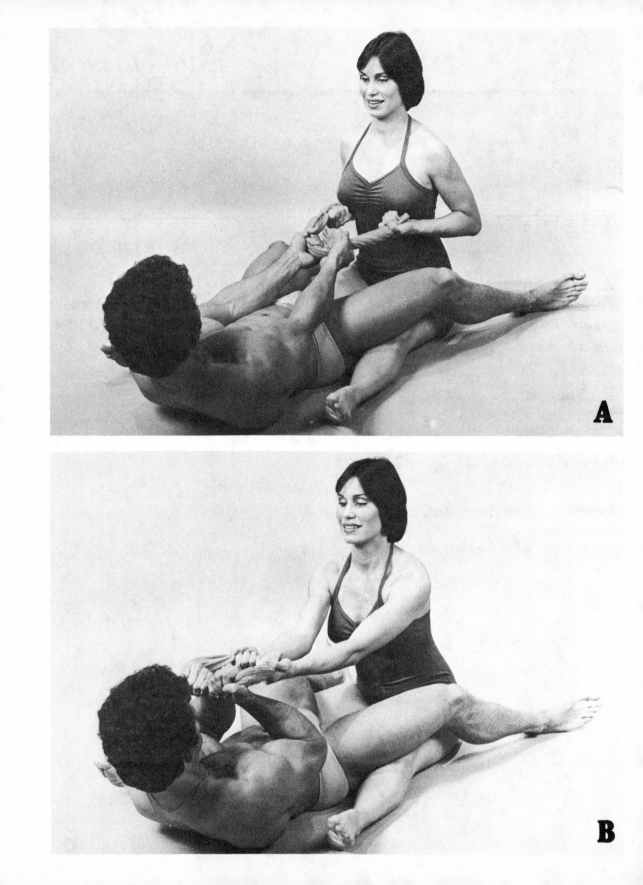

A

B

The Mangle

A *Starting Position.* Sit upright on the floor, legs spread. Partner lies with buttocks between partner's thighs, legs outstretched on either side of partner. Partner grabs the twisted towel at one end and you grab it in the middle. Proceed with tug-of-war.

B Curl your arms up, against partner's resistance, keeping your elbows at your sides.

C Now partner pulls your arms out straight and works against your resistance.

Repetitions: 10 (work up to 20).

Benefits: biceps and wrist, partner's back, arms, and chest muscles.

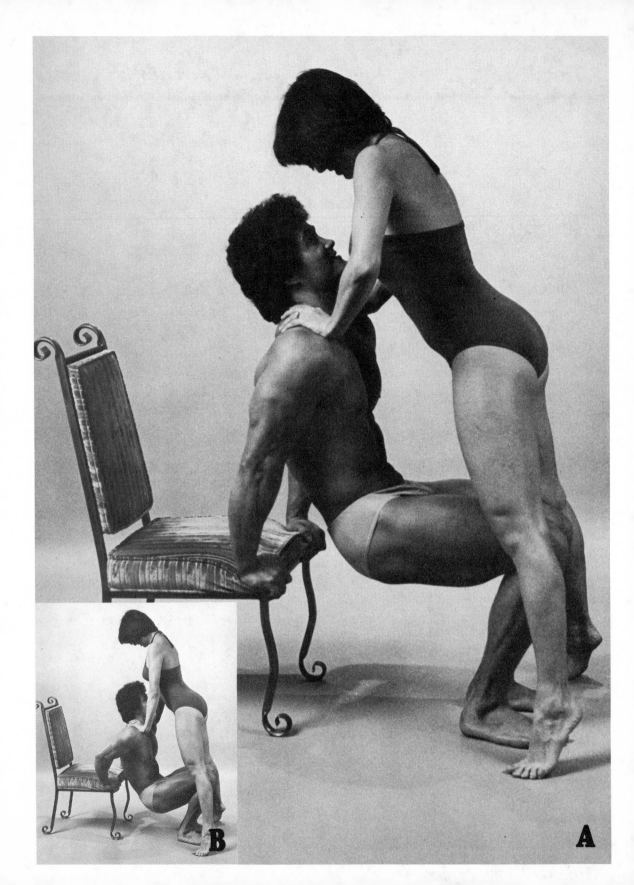

The Washboard

A *Starting Position.* Squat in front of a sturdy chair with your back to the seat, supporting your weight on the palms of your hands. Your partner should stand over you with hands on your shoulders, close to your neck.

B As partner pushes you down, bend your elbows and resist as you go down.

C Push yourself back up using the triceps muscles, while partner resists.

Repetitions: 10 (work up to 20).

Benefits: triceps, chest, and shoulder muscles, and partner's chest and arm muscles.

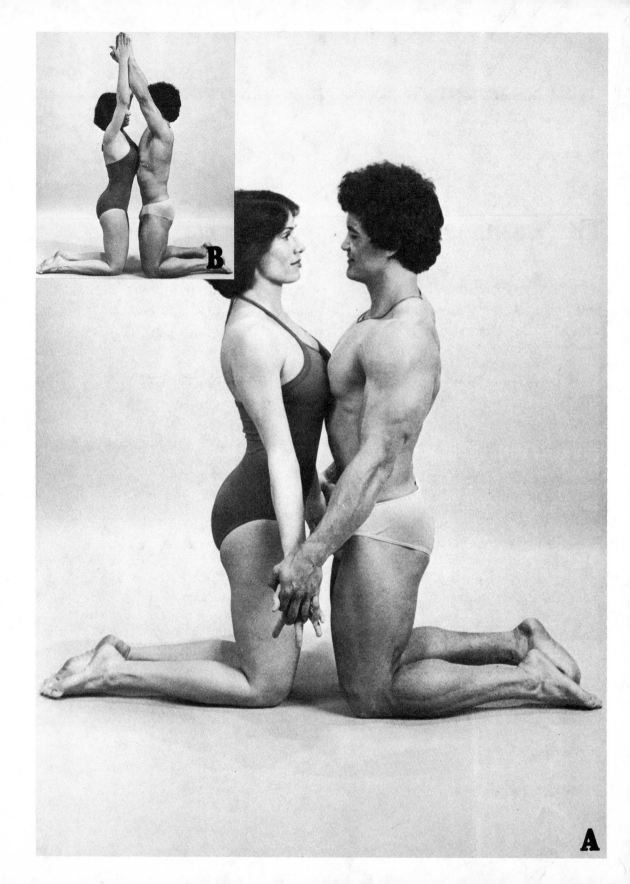

The Double Semaphore

A *Starting Position.* Kneel upright with your chests touching, arms down, your hands on top of partner's hands, palms are up, fingers extended.

B Partner raises arms sideways and up, as you push down, elbows locked.

C Push partner's arms down against resistance, elbows locked.

Repetitions: 10 (work up to 20).

Benefits: shoulder and back muscles.

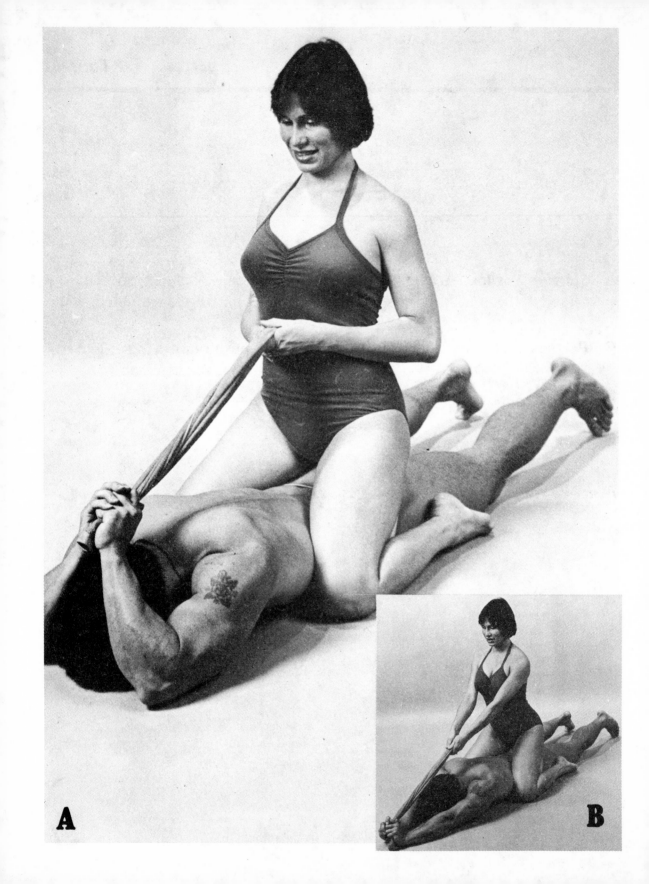

A

B

Dolphin Ride

A *Starting Position.* Lie on the floor on your stomach while your partner kneels astraddle of your waist. With your arms bent back at the elbows, hold on to one end of a towel, the partner holds the other end.

B Pull forward without lifting your elbows off the floor, pulling partner's arms forward against resistance.

C As partner pulls back, you resist.

Repetitions: 10 (work up to 20).

Benefits: triceps and forearm muscles and partner's back, chest, and shoulder muscles.

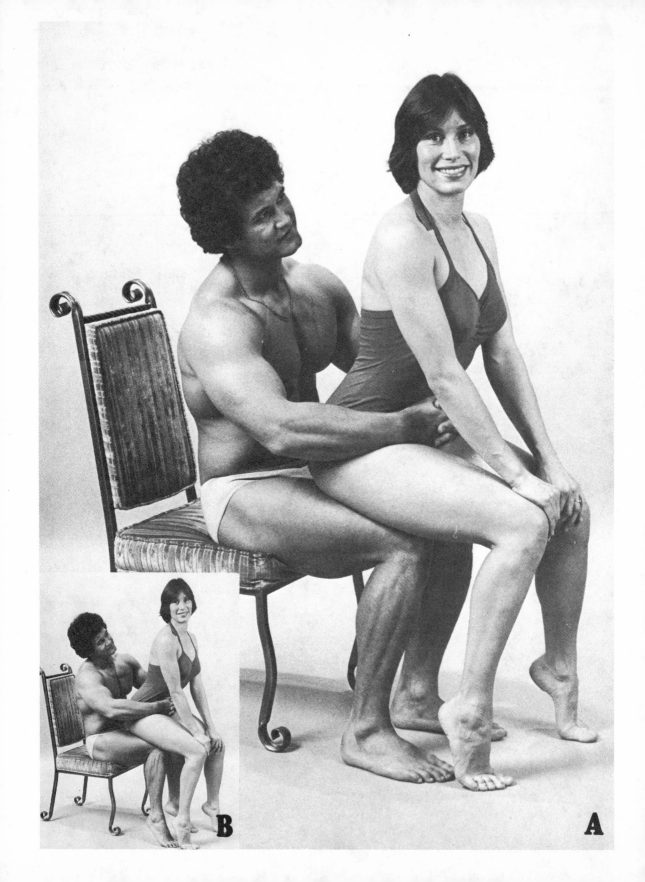

B

A

Joy Ride

A *Starting Position.* One partner sits on the forward half of a chair, and partner sits on your lap, more toward the knee, your arms around partner's waist.

B The sitter raises and lowers his knees, pushing off the toes, and working only the calf muscles.

Repetitions: 15 (work up to 30).

Benefits: calf muscles.

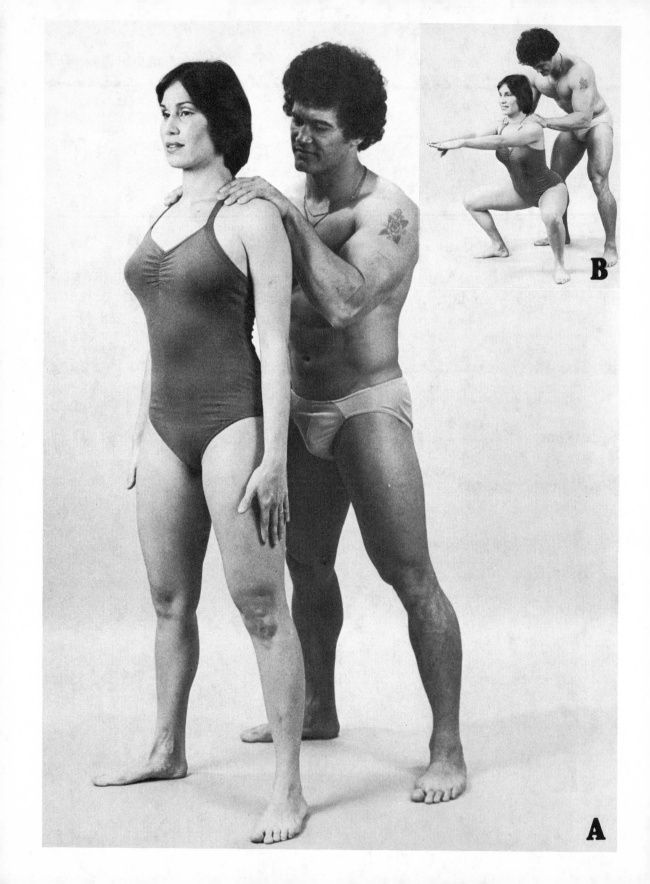

A

B

Heavy-Duty Butter Churn

A *Starting Position.* Partners stand facing each other, legs spread to shoulder width. Hands should be on partner's shoulders, partner's hands at sides.

B Lower yourself into squatting position, bringing your arms forward for balance. Partner will apply pressure as you resist.

C Keep your back straight, and push yourself back up as partner offers resistance by pushing down on your shoulders.

Repetitions: 10 (work up to 20).

Benefits: arms, back, and shoulders and partner's legs.

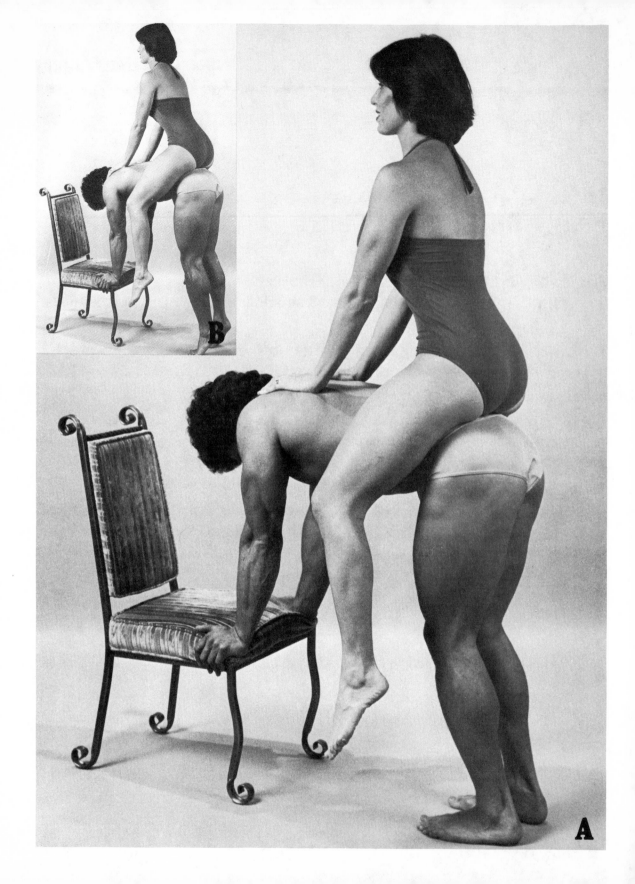

B

A

High Ride

A *Starting Position.* Stand in front of a chair, bent forward at the waist, feet flat on the floor, and grasp the corners of the seat. Partner should sit straddling you as far back on your spine as possible, hands on your back for balance.

B Rise up on toes, then relax.

Repetitions: 15 (work up to 30).

Benefits: calf muscles.

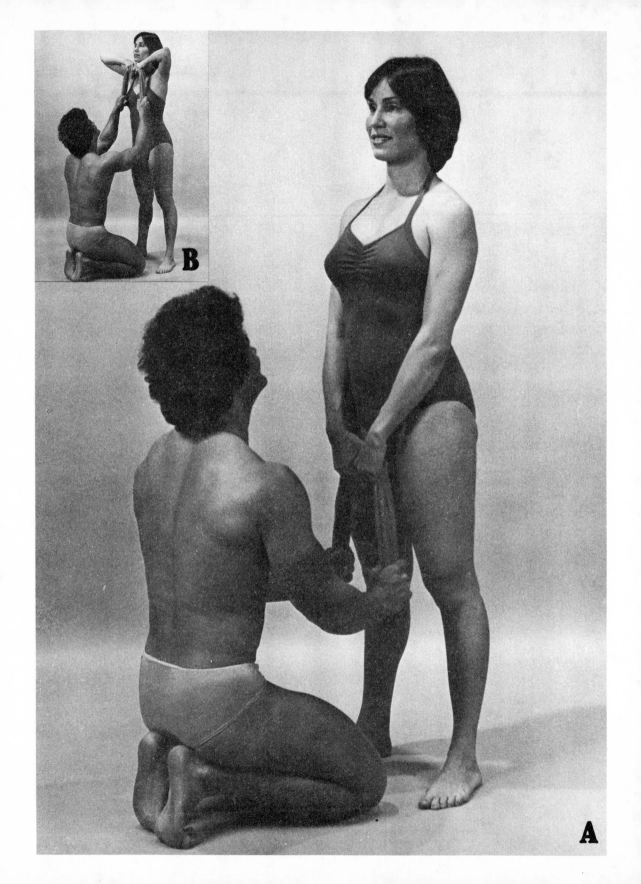

B

A

The Tire Pump

A *Starting Position.* Kneel in front of your partner who should be standing facing you holding the middle of a hand towel, palms inward. Grasp both ends of the towel.

B Keeping hands close to body, partner should raise elbows upward under chin, making sure elbows are high. Resist movement by applying a little pressure.

C Pull down as partner resists. Partner should keep back straight and head high at all times to avoid straining back muscles.

Repetitions: 10 (work up to 20).

Benefits: shoulder, arm, and back muscles and partner's shoulder and arm muscles (especially the trapezius).

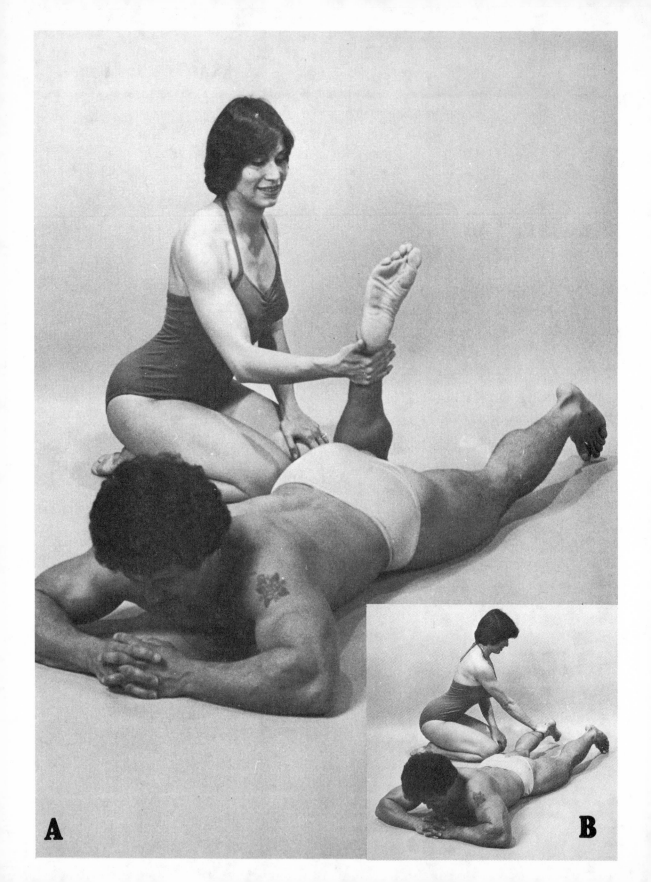

A

B

Paper Cutter

A *Starting Position.* Lie on your stomach on the floor with one leg bent upward at the knee, hands under head, elbows out. Partner kneels beside your upward leg, hands on the back of your heel.

B Partner should push your leg down to the floor as you resist.

C Pull your leg back up again, while partner resists.

Repetitions: 10 (work up to 20).

Benefits: leg biceps and partner's arm and chest muscles.

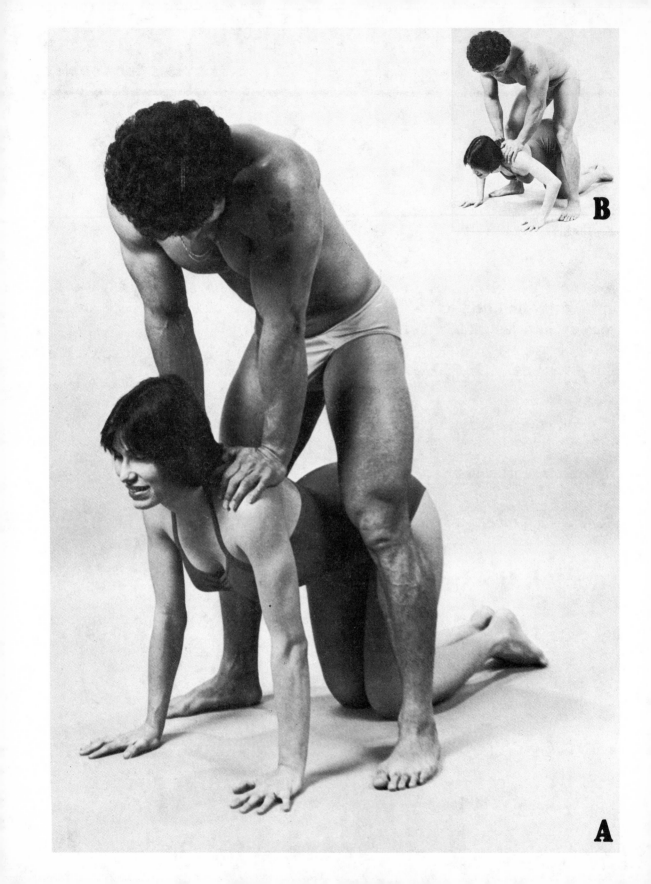

A

B

The Pusher

A *Starting Position.* Get on your hands and knees, with partner standing over you straddling your waist, with hands on your shoulders.

B Partner pushes down as you bend your elbows and offers resistance going down.

C Push yourself back up while partner resists with a little pressure. Start with little resistance and work up to more, slowly.

Repetitions: 10 (work up to 20).

Benefits: chest muscles and partner's back and arm muscles.

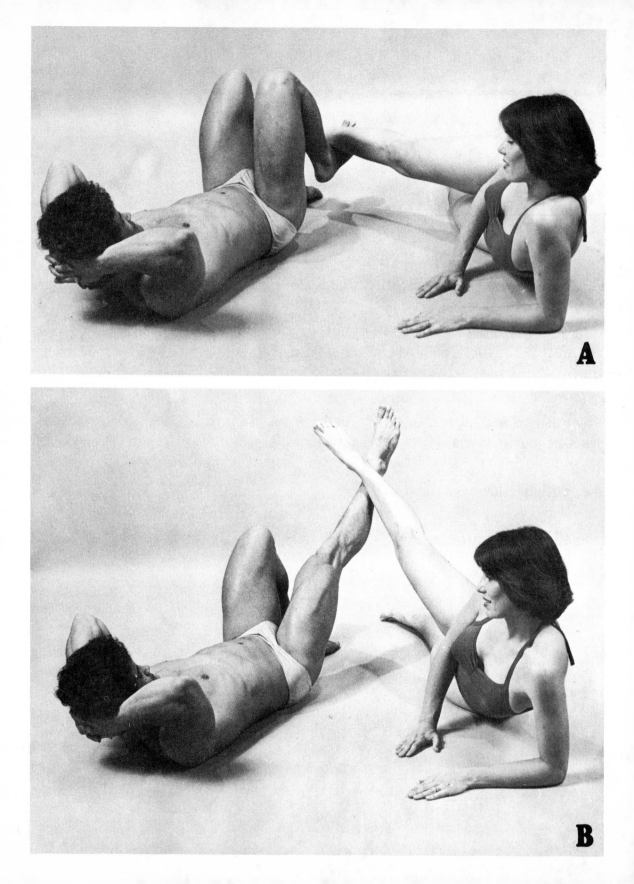

Can-Can Kick

A *Starting Position.* Lie on your back, knees up, hands behind head with fingers interlocked, head up, and the right foot off the floor about four to six inches. Partner should lie on left side diagonally beside you, right calf resting on your upraised right foot.

B Extend your left leg forward and upward. Partner's leg is only for added weight, no resistance is needed.

C Partner pushes your leg back down as you resist. Both partners change sides and repeat.

Repetitions: 10 (work up to 20).

Benefits: legs, stomach muscles, and partner's inner thighs.

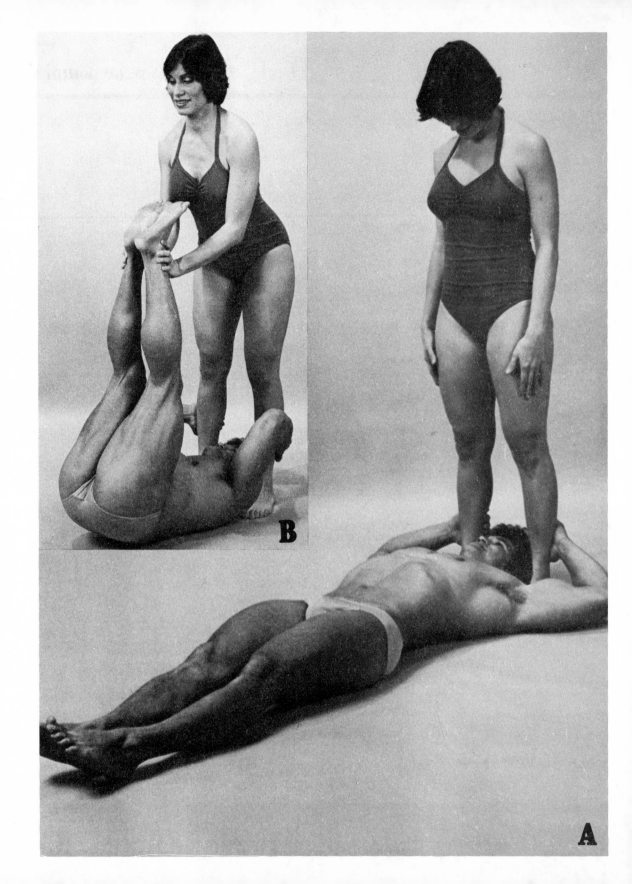

B

A

Leg Bopper

A *Starting Position.* Lie on your back and grasp your partner's ankles or legs, as partner stands straddling your head.

B Keeping your knees locked and feet together, raise your legs swiftly.

C Your partner catches your ankles and gives a strong push to send your legs down again. The motion should be very fast.

Repetitions: 10 (work up to 30).

Benefits: stomach muscles, and partner's shoulder, arm, and back muscles.

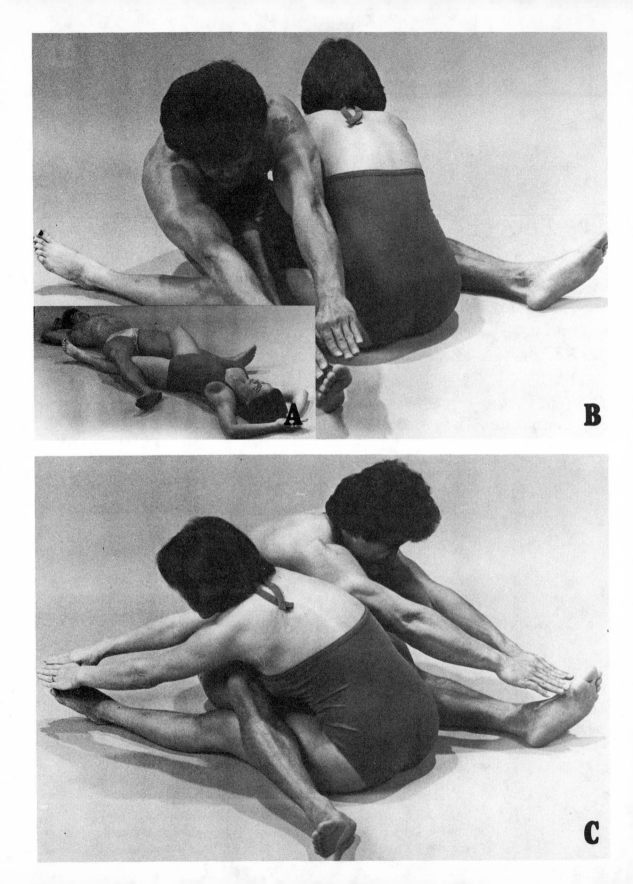

The Cross Road

A *Starting Position.* Both partners lie on their backs with legs entwined: Your right thigh atop partner's left calf, partner's right calf over your left thigh. Hands over head, legs spread far apart.

B Simultaneously sit-up touching your right toes with both hands.

C Partners return to starting position, then repeat touching the opposite toes. Reverse directions with each sit-up.

Repetitions: 10 (work up to 20).

Benefits: stomach muscles.

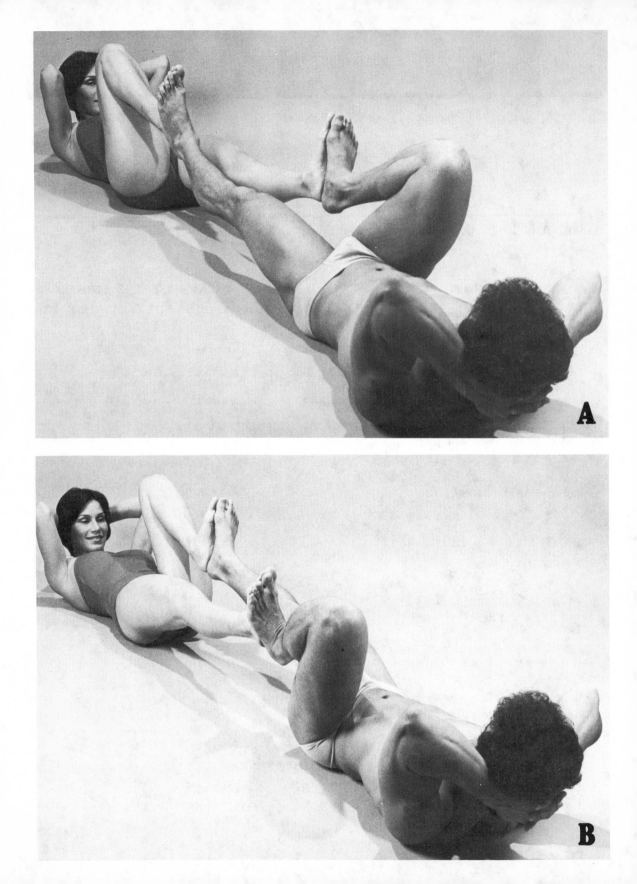

A

B

Choo-Choo Train

A *Starting Position.* Both partners lie on their backs, legs off the floor, one leg drawn up toward the chest, the other extended with soles of the feet together. Hands should be behind raised head, fingers interlocked. Head should be up at all times.

B Keeping the soles of your feet tightly together, extend one leg then the other leg forcing the partner's leg backward. Change legs with each motion. Get a steady motion going.

Repetitions: 10 (work up to 20).

Benefits: leg and stomach muscles.

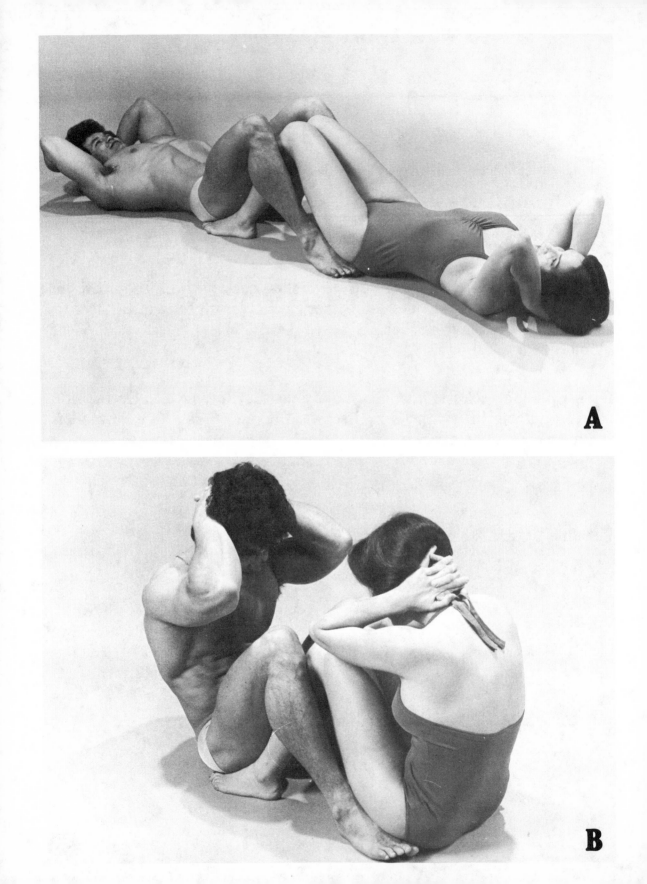

A

B

Bookends

A *Starting Position.* Both partners lie on their backs, with feet on the outside and slightly under the other partner's buttocks, one set of knees inside the other partner's knees. Hands should be behind heads, fingers interlocked, and elbows forward.

B Simultaneously sit-up and touch elbows to knees.

C Lower yourself back down to starting position and repeat.

Repetitions: 10 (work up to 20).

Benefits: stomach muscles of both partners.

CHAPTER 5

Conditioning with the Children

These exercises are designed to be a form of recreation for children, with a little psychological conditioning on the side. You will be doing the work, using the child as a living barbell, with the child going along for the ride. Doing this type of exercise with your children is a means of conditioning them to the idea that exercise is important and enjoyable. They will soon be able to do their own exercises.

Children are highly imaginative, so the exercise experience should be creative as well as beneficial or they will soon be bored with it. They can, however, be too playful, not fully understanding that exercise is a serious business. The parent must patiently instruct the child how to secure the body with the legs and how to make the body rigid or relaxed when required. In the first few sessions make sure the child becomes accustomed to the exercise movements and begins to understand what position the body should be in. When this understanding is reached, the child's imagination can be brought into the exercise.

Involve the child by counting in rhymes. The one we use goes like this: "1-2-3-4 push from the floor; 5-6-7-8 flabby we hate; 1 and 2 me and you; 3 and 4 let's do more; 5 and 6 get your kicks; 7 and 8 don't be late; 9 and 10 now again."

You can also vary the exercise movements to suggest animal movements, carnival rides, playground games or anything the child views as pleasurable and fun. Involve the child for the best experience. Make your exercise sessions a time for total family involvement.

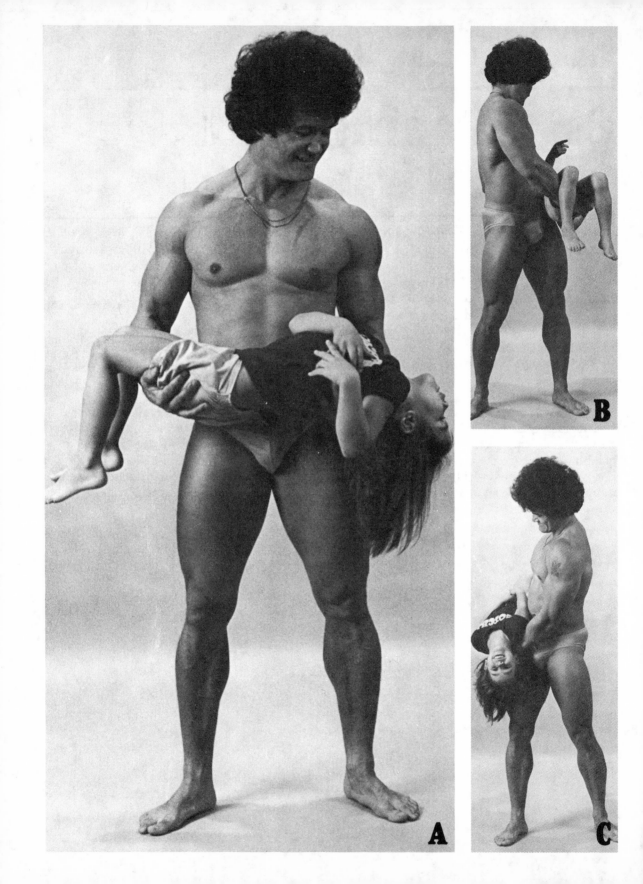

King Kong

A *Starting Position.* Stand in King Kong pose with the child in your arms, and legs spread.

B Swing strongly to the right as far as possible, knees locked, and the lower half stationary.

C Swing strongly to the other side, as far as possible, as in **B**. Continue this movement.

Repetitions: 10 (work up to 20 each side).

Benefits: waist, also a good warm-up exercise.

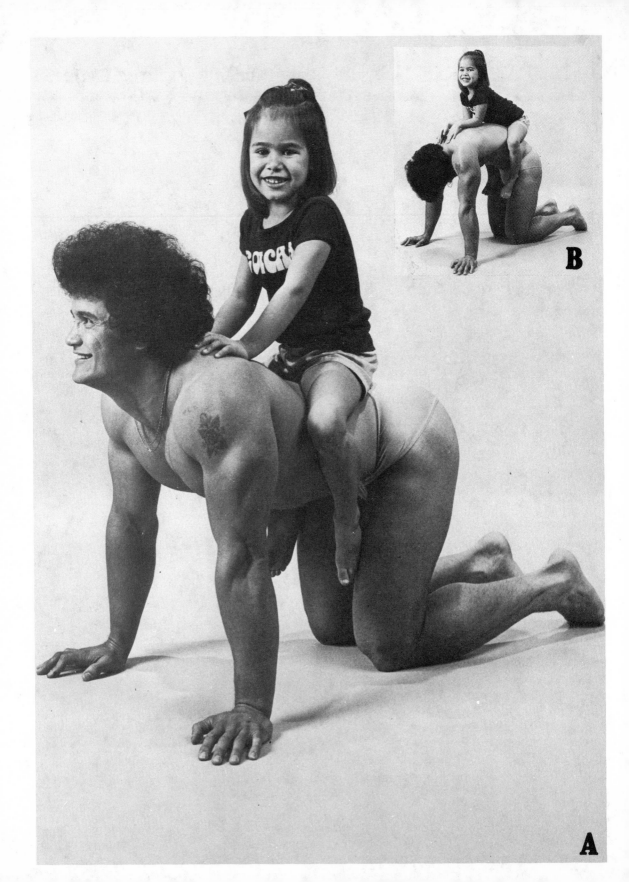

B

A

Bronco Ride

A *Starting Position.* Get on your hands and knees and let the child straddle your mid-back, keep your head up, and relax.

B Arch your back and tuck your head down. You should feel a bunching-up in the stomach.

C Return to the starting position.

Repetitions: 10 (work up to 30).

Benefits: stomach, back, buttocks, and neck muscles.

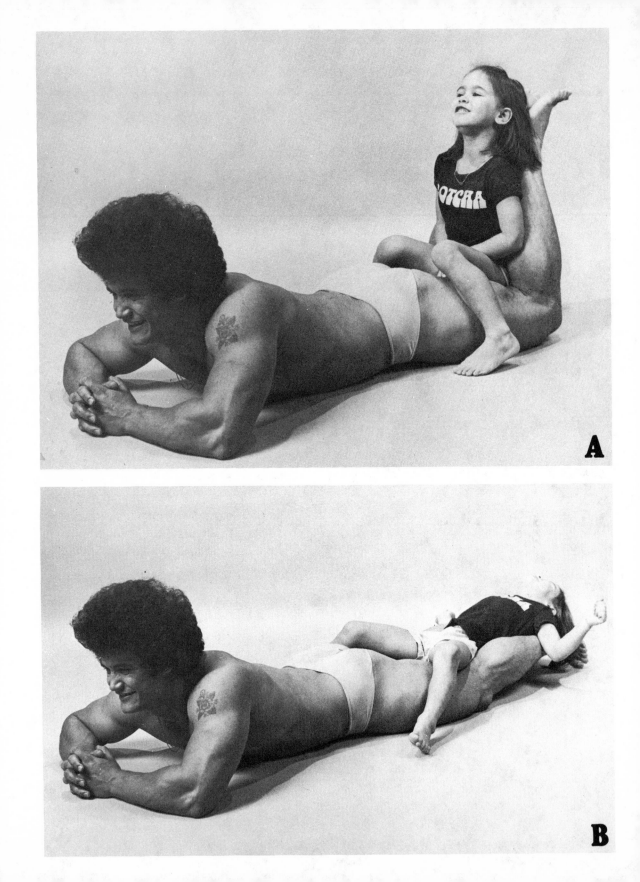

A

B

Rocking Chair

A *Starting Position.* Lie on your stomach with your hands crossed under your chin and your legs bent up at the knees. Keep your legs together. The child should sit on your thighs and lean against your calves with feet on the floor.

B Have the child relax, and go with the movement. Drop your feet down slowly using the muscle on the back of the leg to control the movement. Your feet should go all the way to the floor.

C Raise your feet up again using the muscles in the back of your leg.

Repetitions: 10 (work up to 20).

Benefits: back of the legs, and lower back muscles.

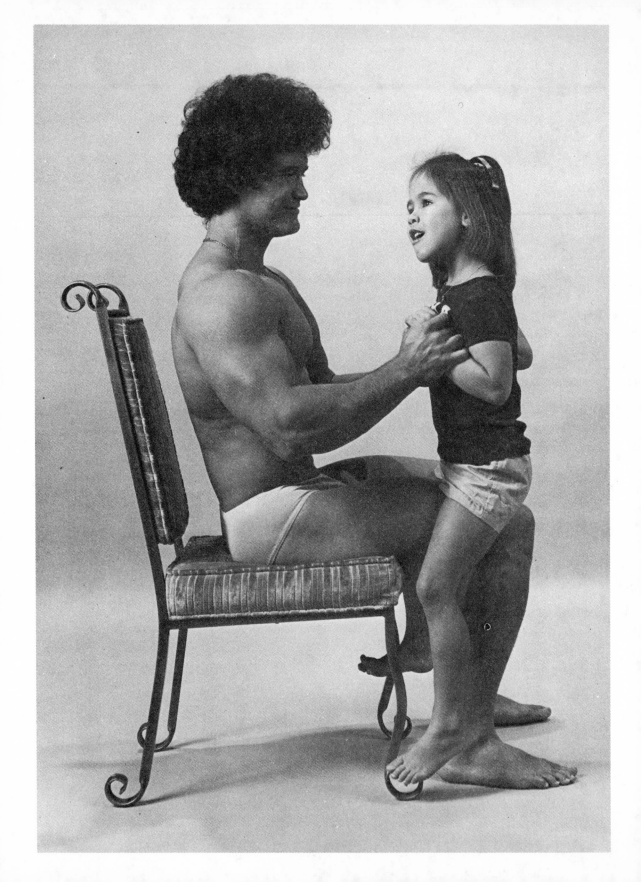

Hobby-Horse

A *Starting Position.* Sit in a chair with your knees together and the child sitting on them facing you.

B With your foot flat on the floor, raise your knee up using the calf muscles to do the work. Lower your foot back down to the starting position.

Repetitions: 10 (work up to 30).

Benefits: calf muscles.

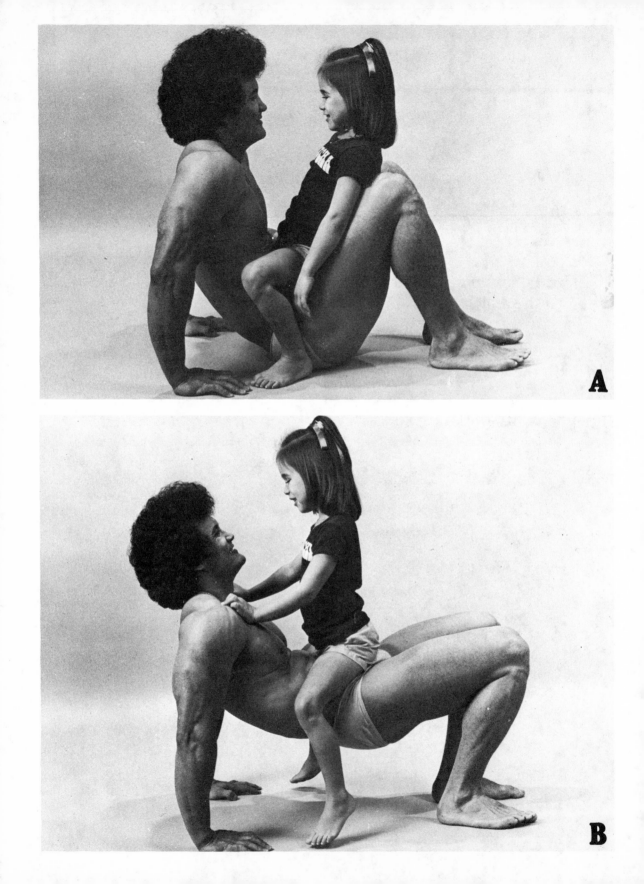

Backward Bronco

A *Starting Position.* Sit on the floor, knees bent up, arms behind you for balance, fingers pointing to the front. (Sag in the middle with the child sitting on your lower abdomen.)

B Raise yourself off the floor on your hands and feet. You should feel a bunching-up in your buttocks.

C Lower yourself back down to the starting position.

Repetitions: 10 (work up to 20).

Benefits: buttocks, leg biceps, triceps, back, and shoulders.

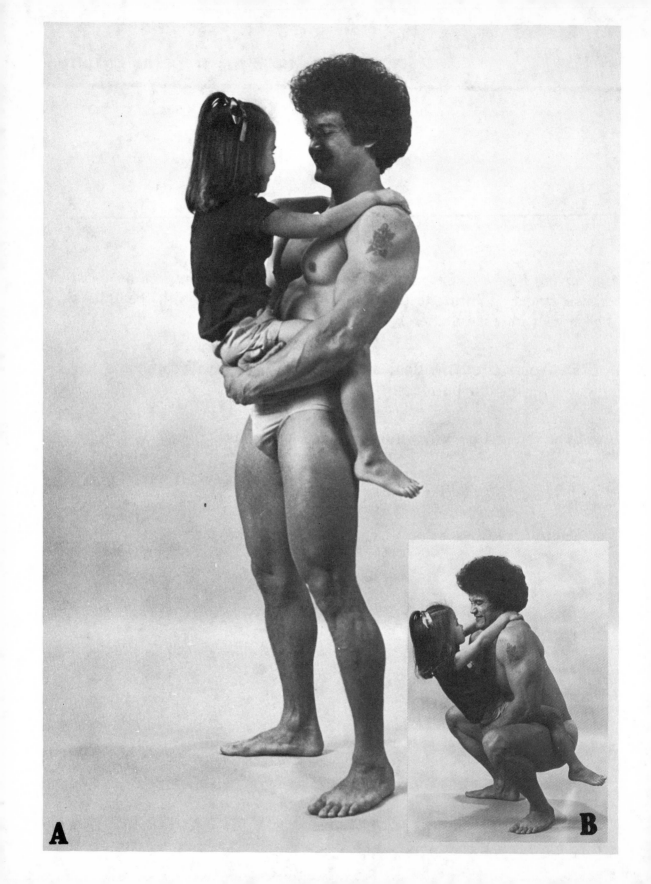

A

B

The Martini

A *Starting Position.* Stand with your feet spread to shoulder width, the child sitting in your clasped arms, facing you with legs hanging through your elbows.

B Using your leg muscles, lower yourself down into a squatting position.

C Push yourself back up to the starting position. The child's legs should move in and out as you go up and down.

Repetitions: 6 (work up to 15).

Benefits: leg and buttocks muscles.

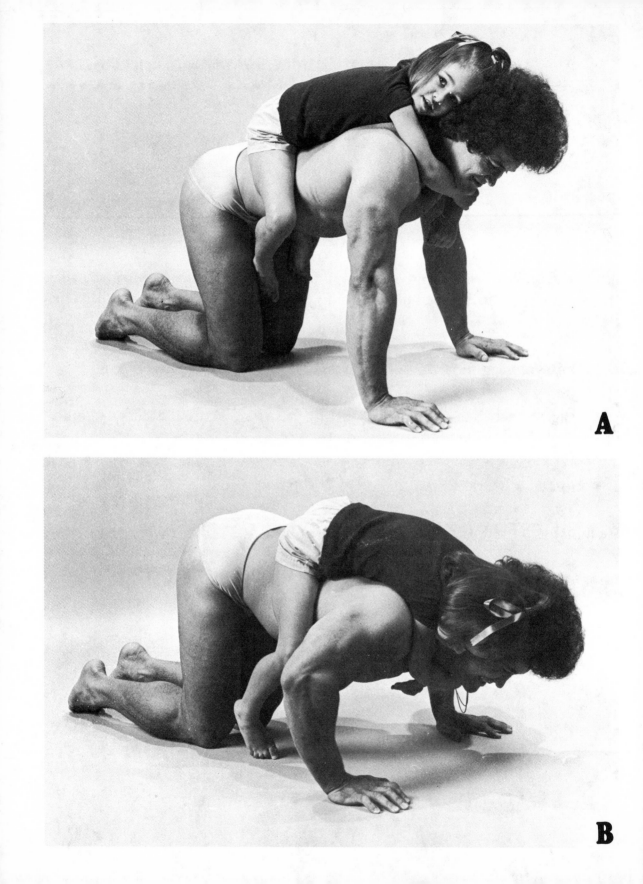

A

B

Turtle-Ride

A *Starting Position.* Get into a push-up position, arms spread wider than shoulder width. Have the child wrap both legs around your waist, arms around your neck.

B Bend at the elbow, lower your chest toward the floor.

C Using the chest muscles, push yourself back up.

Repetitions: 6 (work up to 12).

Benefits: chest and arms.

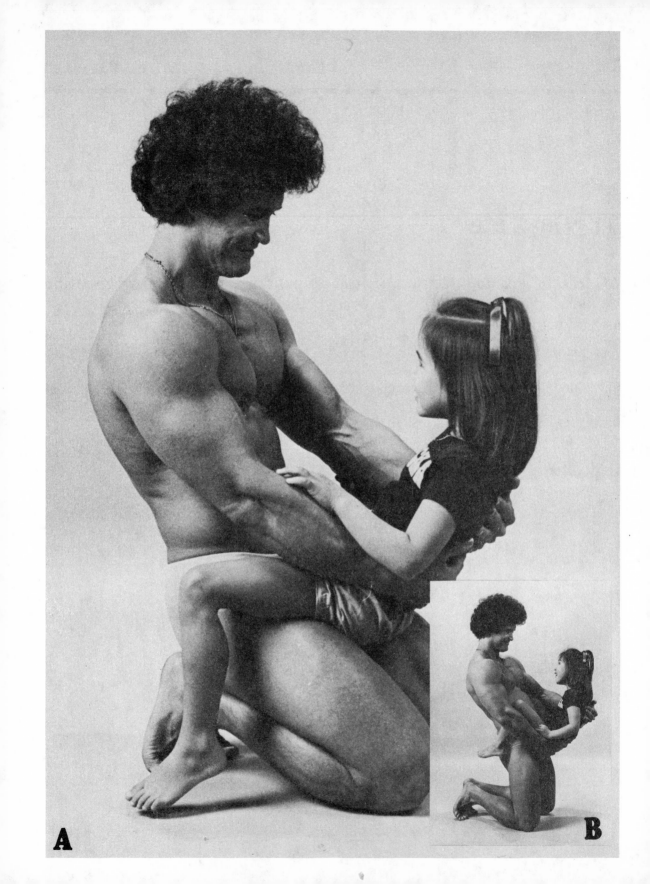

A

B

The Swings

A *Starting Position.* Kneel on the floor, sitting on your heels. Hold the child in a comfortable position against your chest, legs around your waist.

B Raise up, thrusting your pelvis forward, from the kneeling position.

C Bring yourself back to the starting position.

Repetitions: 10 (work up to 20).

Benefits: thigh, buttocks, and abdominal muscles.

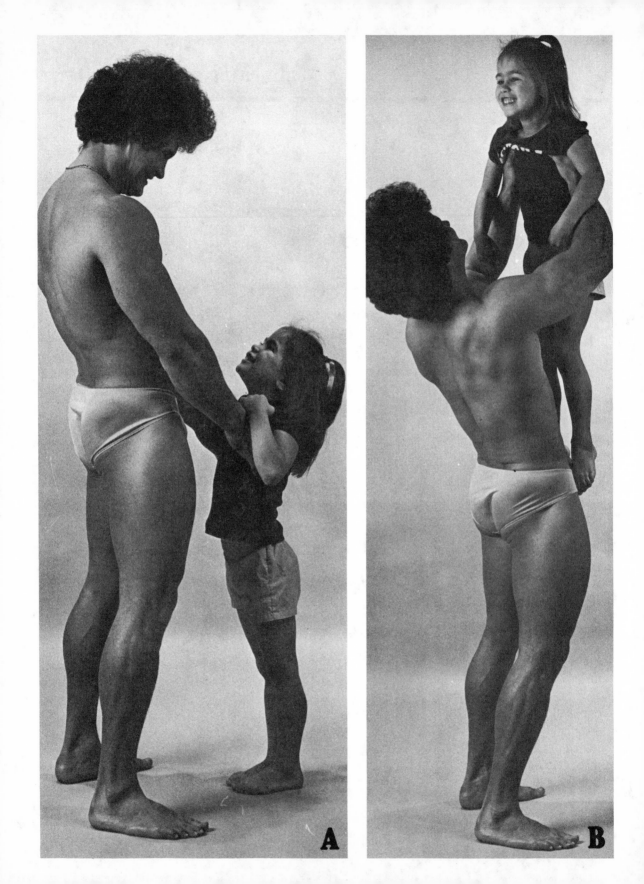

The Giggle Machine

A *Starting Position.* Stand with your feet at shoulder width. Grab the child under her arms.

B Using the shoulder muscle, lift the child straight up above your head.

C Lower the child back down to the floor. You should have the child bend her knees to the bottom and push off on the rise.

Repetitions: 10 (work up to 15).

Benefits: back, chest, shoulder, and arm muscles.

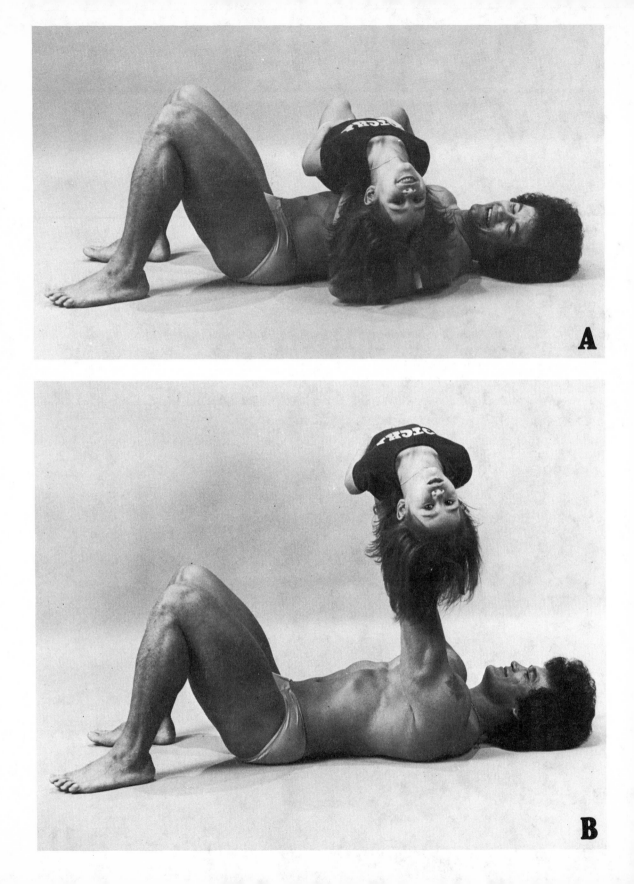

A

B

Low-Rider

A *Starting Position.* Lie on your back, knees drawn up, and hold the child in your hands, one hand by the neck and back area, the other hand under the knee area, your upper arms and elbow flat on the floor.

B Using the chest muscles, push the child up, arms extended.

C Lower the child back to the starting position.

Repetitions: 10 (work up to 20).

Benefits: arm and chest muscle.

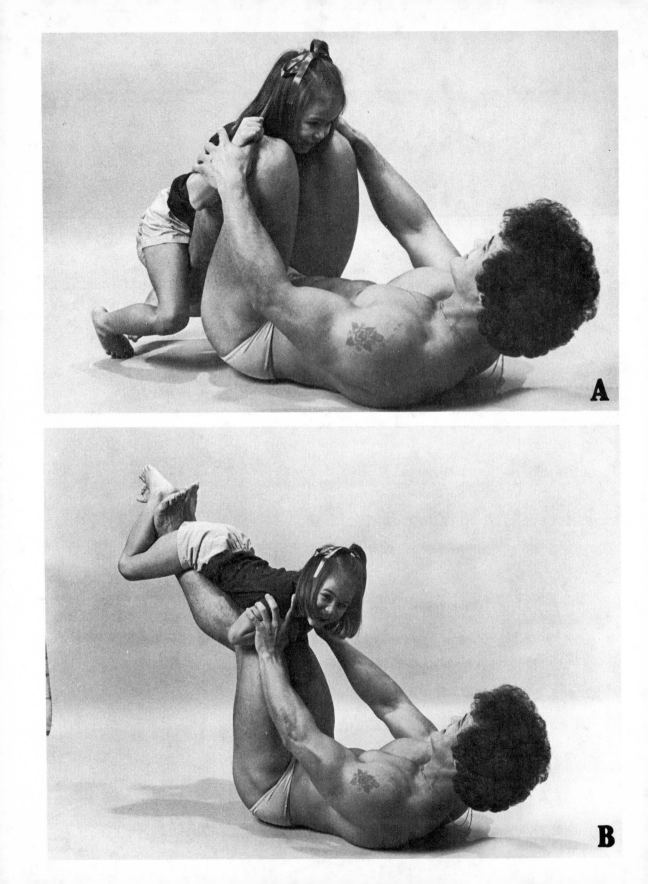

See-Saw

A *Starting Position.* Lie on your back with your knees drawn up and toes turned in. With your hands around the child's shoulders, have her sit on the tops of your feet with her chest against your shins.

B Extend your lower leg forward and upward. Go slowly at first, and hold the child in place by grasping the shoulder area.

C Lower your upper leg back to the starting position.

Repetitions: 5 (work up to 15).

Benefits: leg, abdominal, and back muscles.

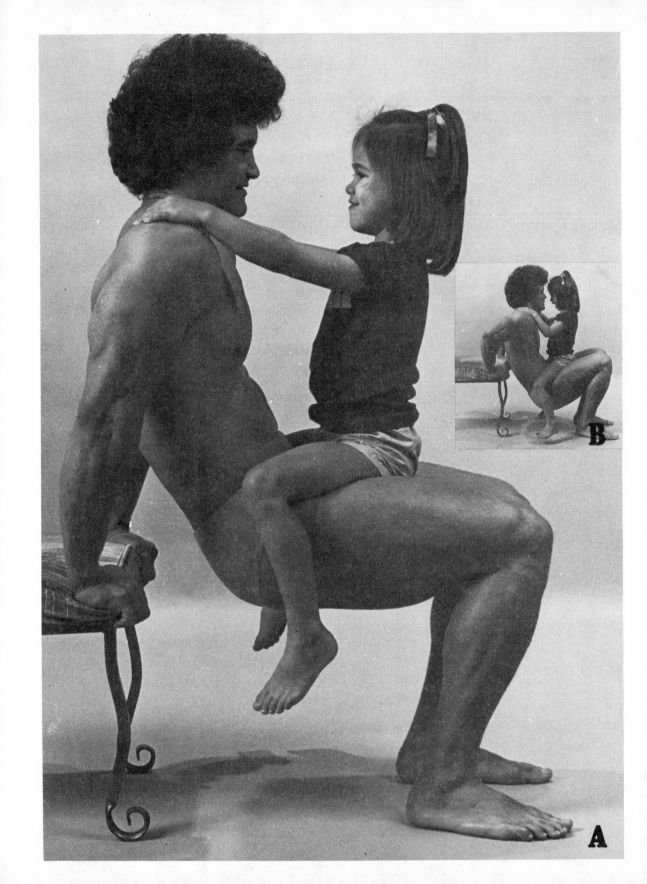

The Kiddy Cantilever

A *Starting Position.* Place a sturdy chair against the wall. Squat in front of it. With the palms of your hands behind you, support your weight on the very front of the chair. Have the child sit in the sag of your lower abdomen, holding on to your shoulders.

B Lower your buttocks to the floor by bending at the elbow and using your triceps muscles to do the work.

C Push back up into the starting position.

Repetitions: 10 (work up to 15).

Benefits: back of the arm (triceps), chest, and shoulders.

PART 2

EXERCISES FOR SPECIAL TIMES

CHAPTER 6

Pregnancy Exercises

Why exercise during pregnancy? There are several reasons why a regular program of exercises is important during pregnancy. The first is that it aids and improves blood circulation, which is all-important during pregnancy. The second is that it tones and controls your muscles, a vital process during labor and delivery.

Finally, you will find that with your muscles strong and toned, you will carry your child with more ease and comfort. You will not sag so much or feel so burdened as you enter the final stages of your pregnancy—and throughout the entire experience you will have more energy. (It is a curious axiom of exercise that the more energy you expend, the more you will have in reserve.)

There are several systems of exercises (most notably the Lamaze) that are specifically designed to develop control in the muscles used in giving birth. This system is not that specific in purpose. It is designed as a supplement. The exercises keep the body limber and supple and provide good muscle tone for an easier delivery.

In addition, the exercises will help you burn off unwanted calories, and by getting you into good condition before the birth, will help your body recuperate faster afterward.

The general feeling of health and well-being that you will derive from exercising is perhaps one of the greatest benefits to be gained.

A few general rules for beginning an exercise program during pregnancy follow:

1. Always begin working out slowly, picking up the pace as you go along. Don't plunge right in, full steam ahead. If your overall health and conditioning are reasonably sound, your pregnancy will not render you in a condition "too delicate" to exercise. (Unless your doctor says differently, of course.)

2. Practice breathing deeply as you do the exercises. Breathing is an important part of all exercise. It especially applies here because proper breathing will be a great help during labor and delivery—as your doctor or midwife will tell you. It is also helpful with the difficult bowel movements that are one of the uncomfortable aspects of the pregnancy.

3. Because the exercises listed here progress in degree of difficulty, we recommend they be started in the order presented. If the last few prove too difficult at first, concentrate on mastering the first few before continuing.

4. Start with the minimum repetitions listed for each exercise and work up to 30, depending on your condition and how you feel. As you become accustomed to doing these exercises, you can do more, but don't push yourself too far. As your pregnancy advances, do only what you can.

5. Consult your medical advisor about undertaking any exercise program. Most women will benefit from this program, but no chance should be taken that it may be harmful to a few.

6. You will be surprised to find that you can continue these exercises even in the advanced stages of pregnancy. If, however, you find you just can't manage easily, ease off. Most normal pregnancies, however, will allow the mother to do most of the exercises well into her ninth month.

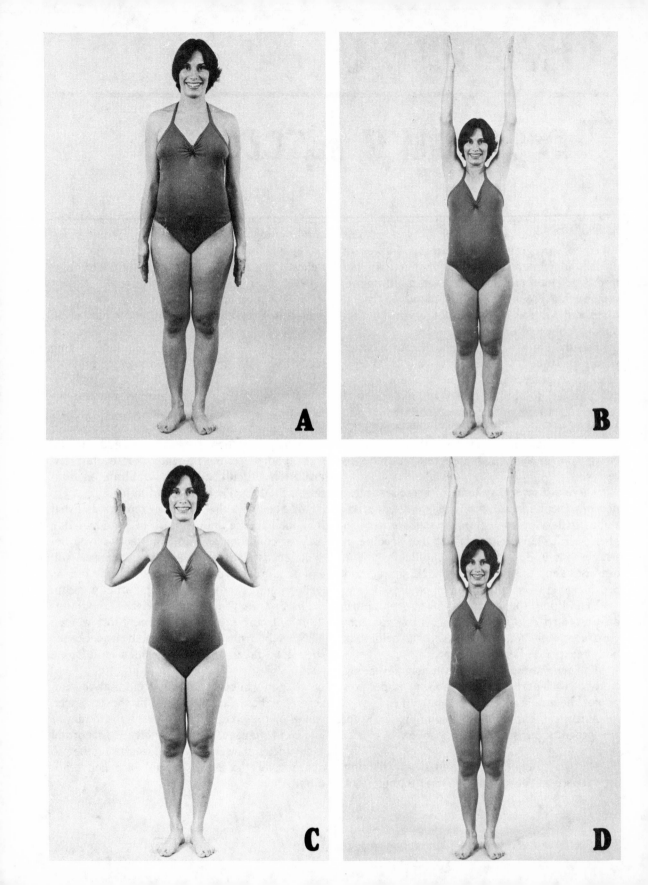

The Semaphore

A *Starting Position.* Stand with your feet a comfortable distance apart, arms at your sides, and shoulders back.

B Locking your elbows, lift your arms straight sideways and upward, palms facing each other.

C Bend your elbows and pull them to your sides, at the same time drawing them back so you feel a bunching-up between your shoulder blades.

D Reach all the way up again. (Don't clap your hands—shoulder-muscle control is important.)

E Drop your hands back to your sides, the same direction as going upward.

Repetitions: 10 (work up to 30).

Benefits: chest, shoulders, upper back, and arms.

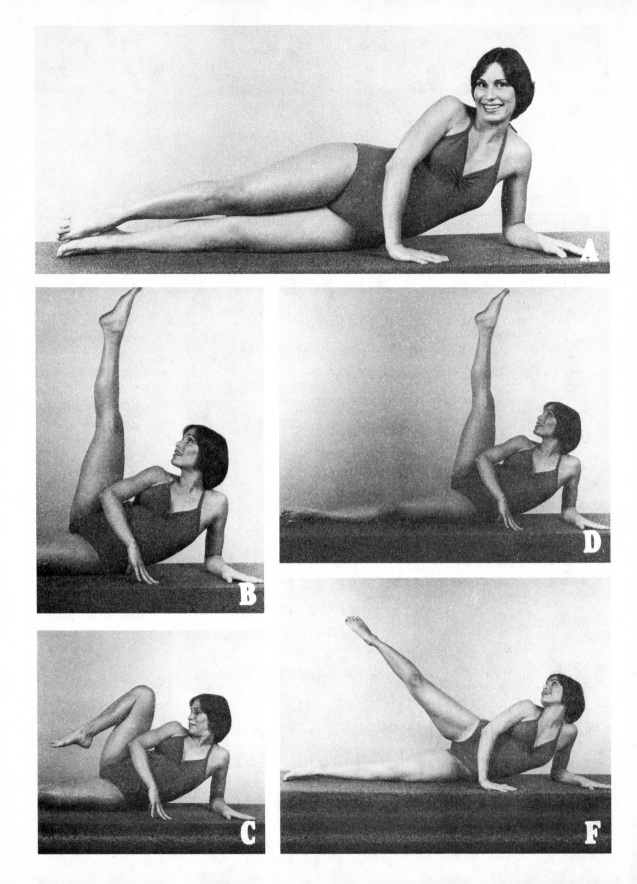

Reclining Ballerina

A *Starting Position.* Lie on your left side with your torso slightly elevated, your weight supported on your left elbow and forearm. Your right arm should be over in front of you, for balance, resting lightly on the floor.

B Lift your right leg up (locking knee straight) as far as you can and rotate your foot so the toe points over your head. Do not strain your muscles by trying to go too high, too soon.

C At the top of your kick, bend your knee lowering your lower leg down as far as it can go.

D Straighten it to the high kick position.

E Lower leg back to the starting position.

F Rotate your hips forward taking your weight on your left forearm and right hand. Kick diagonally to the rear, looking toward your heel, and keep knee locked.

G Bring your leg back to the starting position. Repeat exercise lying on right side.

Repetitions: 6 (work up to 15 each side).

Benefits: midriff, waist, hips, buttocks, and thighs.

125

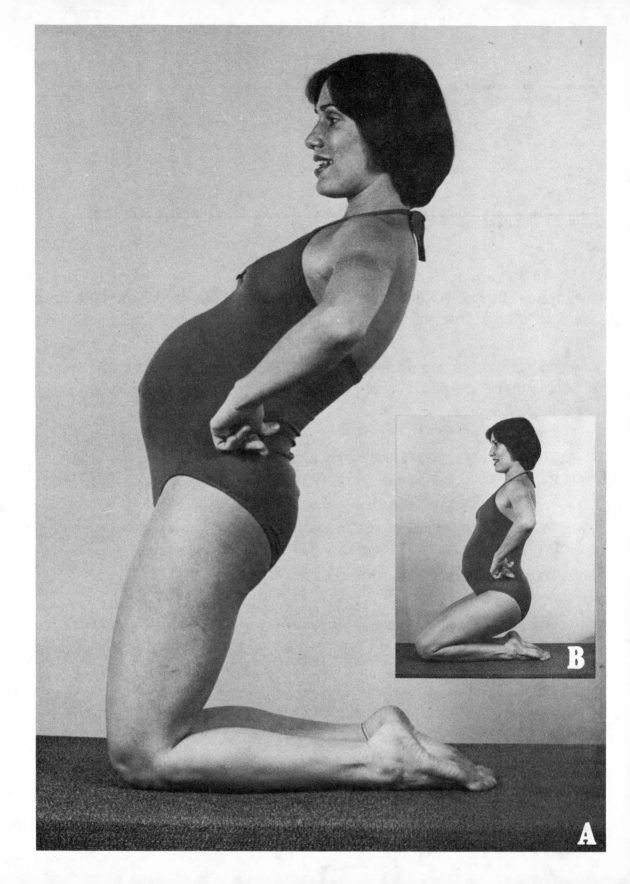

B

A

Rock-a-bye Baby

A *Starting Position.* Kneel and sit back on your heels with feet pointed. Cross your arms across your stomach or on your hips. Rock yourself up strongly, thrusting your pelvis forward and upward.

B Rock back again without sitting or putting weight on heels. Repeat.

Repetitions: 15 (work up to 30).

Benefits: thighs, buttocks, and inner thighs.

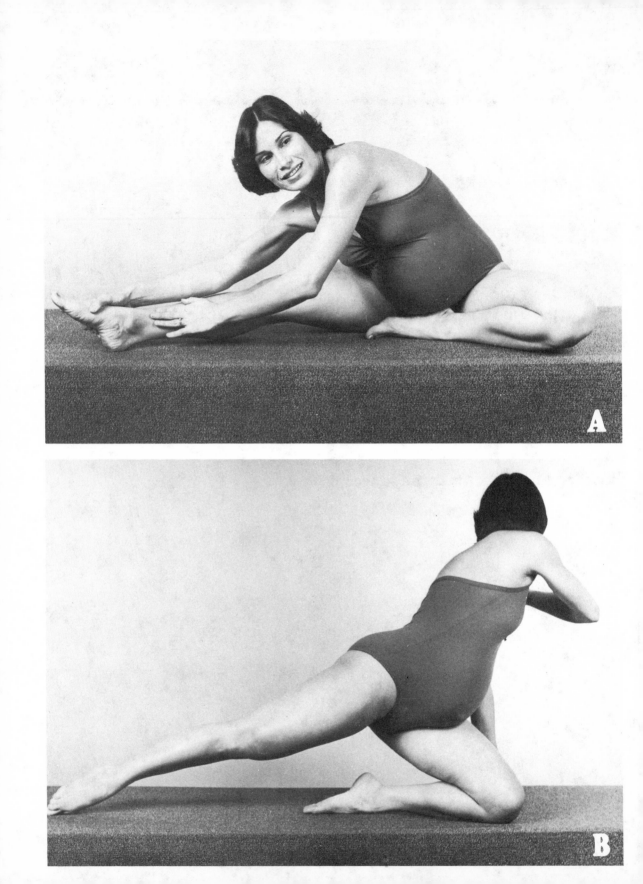

The Side-Car

A *Starting Position.* Get into a kneeling position, knees slightly apart, your arms extended forward, parallel with the floor.

B Sit back and to the side so you sit on one calf, and as you sit you can swing your arms down and to the opposite side, or your hands can remain extended.

C Reverse motion to the other side.

Repetitions: 6 alternating side to side (work up to 12).

Benefits: stomach and leg muscles.

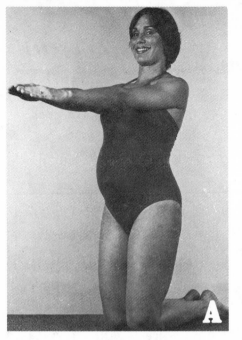

A

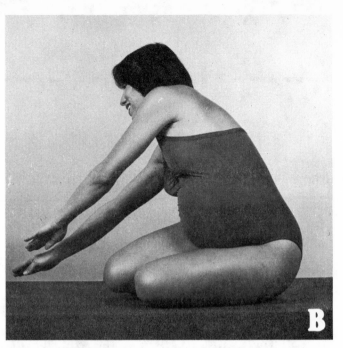

B

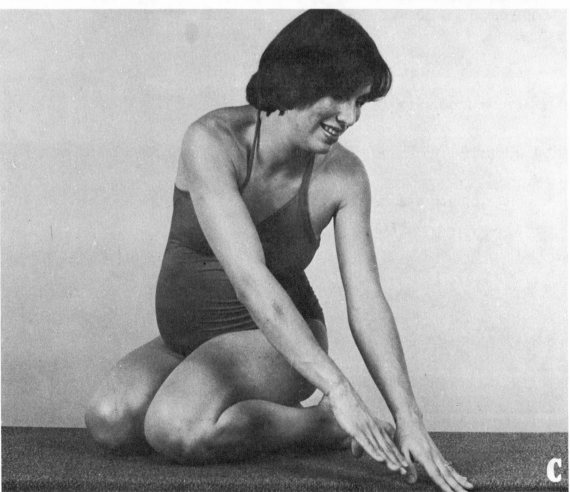

C

The Flying Half-Lotus

A *Starting Position.* Sit on the floor and spread your legs as far as possible, tucking your left heel into your crotch. Your right leg should be straight out to the side with knee locked.

B Grab your right foot with your right hand and touch your right ankle with left hand.

C Bring your left hand back onto the floor next to the left thigh and push yourself up lifting your hips up off the floor. At the same time swinging your right arm around and up, over to the left. As you do this, twist your head and upper body to the left, looking at your heel.

D Reverse the motion, lowering yourself back to the starting position.

Repetitions: 6 (work up to 15 each side).

Benefits: leg muscles, pelvic area, waist and back up the spinal column, shoulders, neck, and arms.*

*Until you are accustomed to stretching, you might feel a strong pulling sensation in the lower abdominal muscles and lower back. If there is any resulting discomfort, stop the exercise immediately.

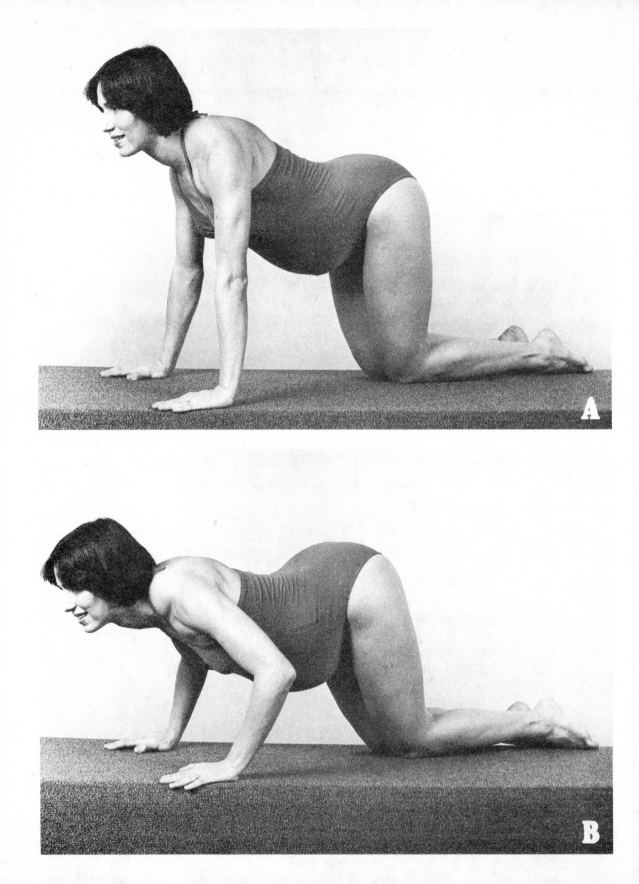

Washer-Woman

A *Starting Position.* Get on your hands and knees, knees together, arms a little wider than shoulder-width, your head up at all times.

B Do a modified push-up, bending at the elbows. Only go down about a fourth of the way at first, and as your strength increases, go lower.

C Push yourself back to the starting position using your chest muscle.

Repetitions: 8 (work up to 20).

Benefits: chest, arm, and upper back muscles.

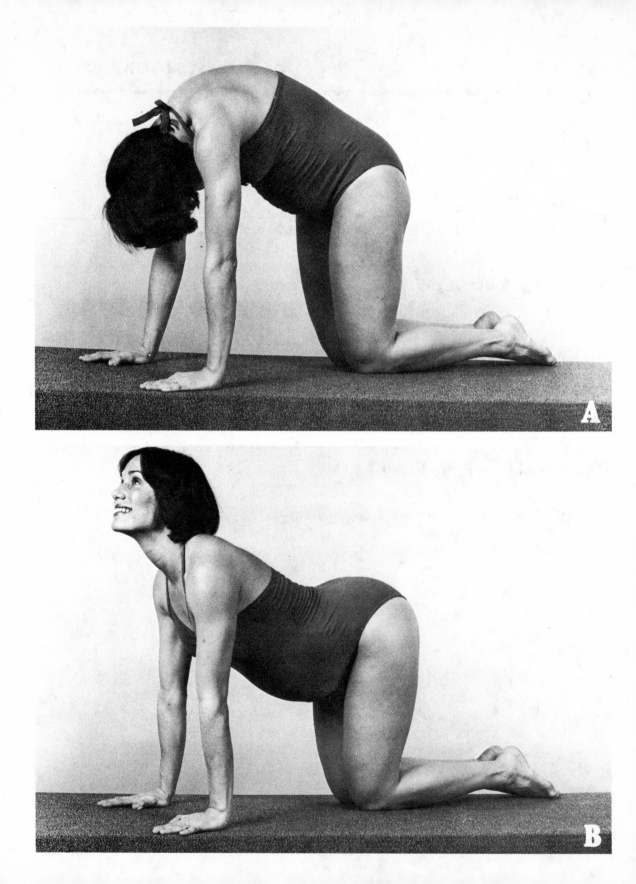

Lady Bronco

A *Starting Position.* Get on your hands and knees, knees slightly apart, arms a little wider than shoulder-width. Put your palms flat on the floor. Hunch up your back and drop your head between your arms and pull your stomach up as tightly as you can.

B Hold until you get maximum tightness, then release, bringing your head up and arching your back. Repeat.

Repetitions: 10 (work up to 30).

Benefits: stomach, back, and neck muscles.

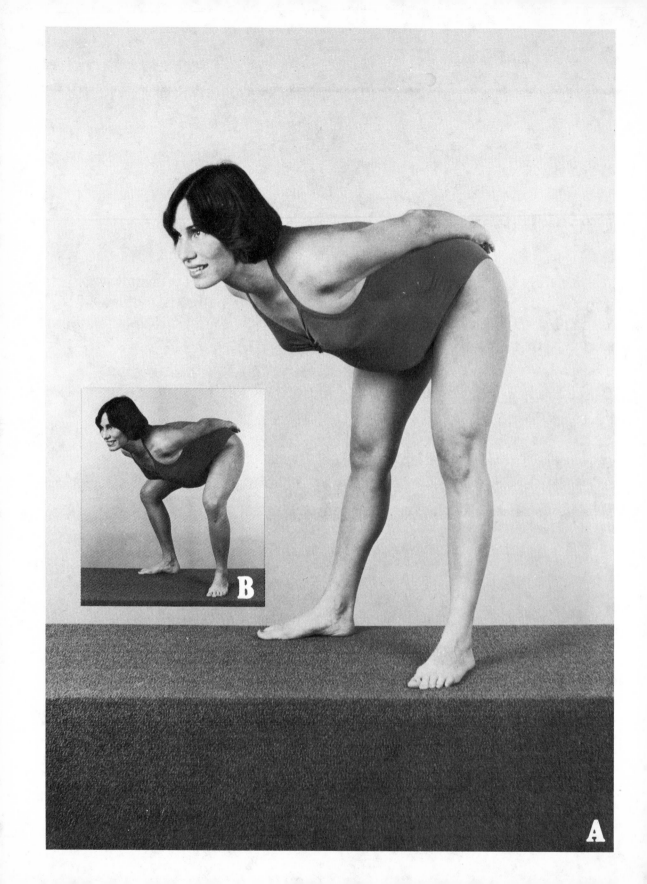

B

A

The Earth Mother

A *Starting Position.* Stand with your legs spread to shoulder-width, toes pointed out, body bent forward at the waist at a forty-five degree angle, hands clasped behind your back, and head up.

B Squat as far down as possible, bending your knees outward, head up.

C Push yourself up to the starting position using leg muscles.

Repetitions: 10 (work up to 30).

Benefits: inner thighs right up into vaginal area, buttocks, and calves.

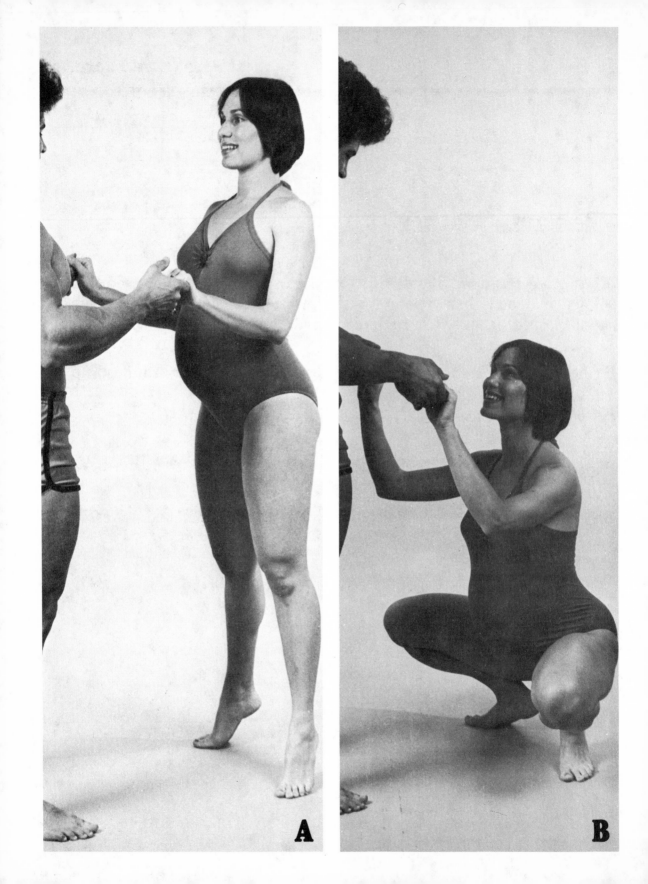

A

B

Tippy Toe Squats

A *Starting Position.* Stand on your tiptoes (toes pointed out) with your feet at a forty-five degree angle, holding onto your partner's forearm or a door frame.

B Squat down, bending your knees out as far as possible. Do not hold at the bottom of the squat.

C Push yourself forward and up to the starting position. Go up and down in a regular rhythm and stay on your toes.

Repetitions: 10 (work up to 30).

Benefits: lower and upper leg, and inner thigh muscles.

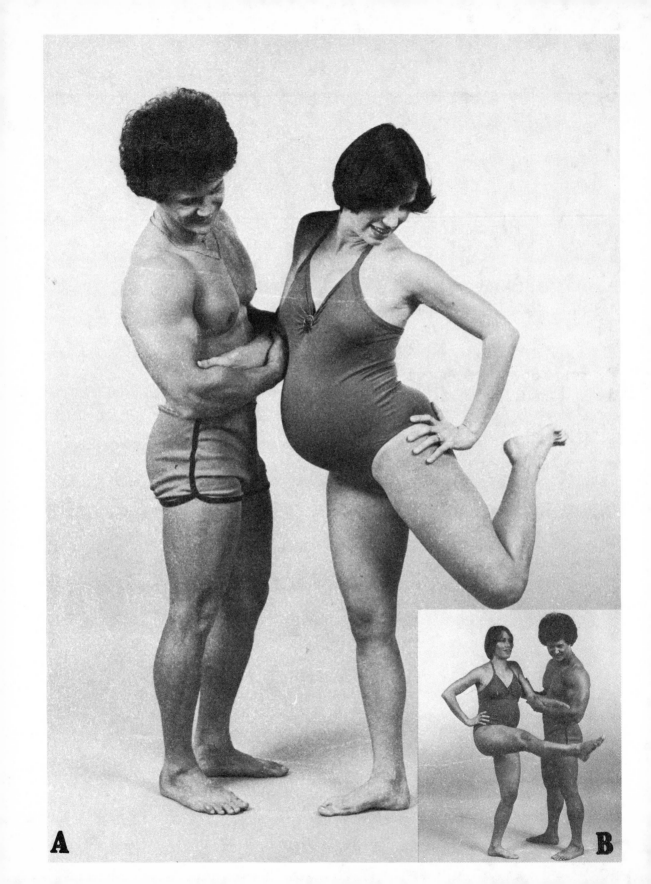

A

B

High Punt Kick

A *Starting Position.* Hold onto partner's forearm or door frame and stand on one foot in a comfortable position.

B Curl the raised foot under your buttocks, push your knees back, arch your back, and look at your foot.

C Kick your curled foot forward and upward, toe pointed.

D Bring your foot back to the curl position in a smooth motion. Reverse position and repeat.

Repetitions: 10 (work up to 15 on each side).

Benefits: leg, stomach, and back muscles.

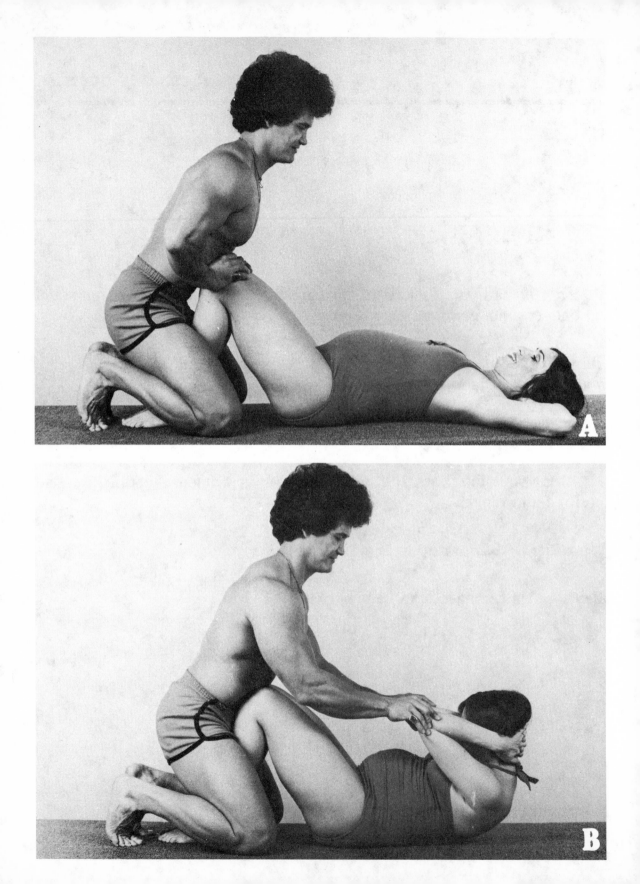

Infant Crunch

A *Starting Position.* Lie on your back with your knees up and feet on the floor, your hands folded under your head. Your partner should squat in front of you, with arms around your upraised knees.

B Bring your elbows close together in front of your face, curl up as far forward as you can, keeping the small of back on the floor. Count four to curl up.

C Count another four as you hold at the top of your curl.

D Count four more as you uncurl back to the starting position.

Repetitions: 6 (work up to 12).

Benefits: stomach muscles used during labor and delivery.

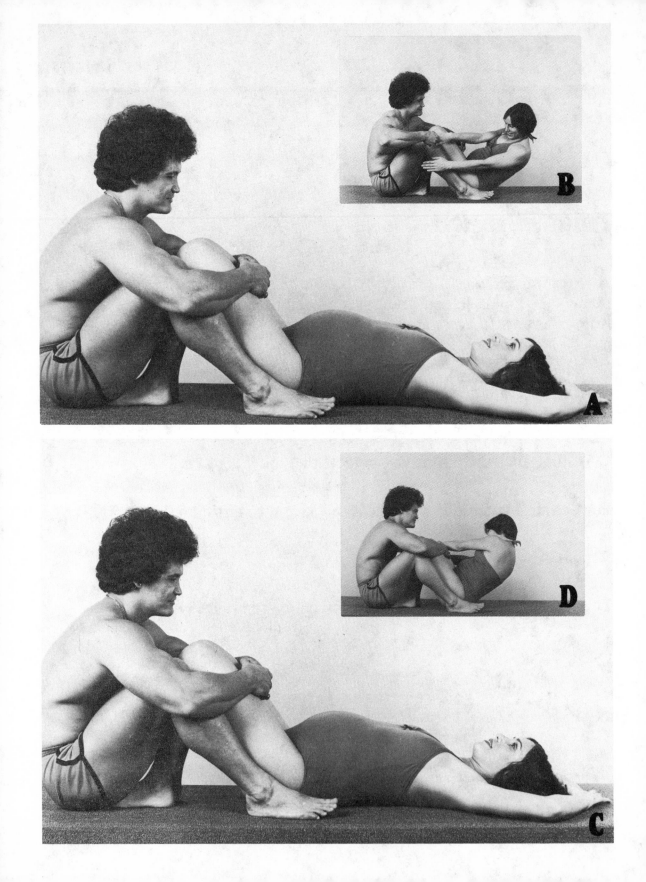

Expulsion Curl-Ups

A *Starting Position.* Lie on your back with your knees up, feet on the floor, arms stretched overhead. Your partner should squat in front of you, with arms folded around your upraised knees.

B Come up straight from the hips, reaching forward and to the right side, twisting your shoulders and upper body to the right. Turn and touch the floor beside your right ankle. Take four counts to get yourself to the touching point.

C Take another four counts to reverse back to the starting position.

D Repeat exercise on the opposite side.

Repetitions: 6 (work up to 12).

Benefits: muscles needed in pushing during contractions and delivery.

CHAPTER 7

Off-Season Athletes

As every person whose profession is dependent upon muscle tone, strength, coordination, and reaction time knows, you cannot let your body get out of shape during the off-season. You must keep those muscles *working efficiently* regardless of your profession. The professional sports participants have a regular pattern of diet and exercise they stick to, even during the off-season. The constant discipline helps keep them in the best physical condition all year round.

The amateur sports participant faces a similar problem. During the summer months a skier has to keep his skiing muscles in shape, and the baseball player has to keep his pitching and hitting muscles in shape during the winter months. You cannot lie around for six months and expect your muscles to respond with the same control and endurance as last season without keeping them in shape.

Included here are 8 special exercises to work you a little harder than your Daily Dozen and in several different areas. They are designed to keep the off-season sports participant in top competitive shape. The intention here is not to build muscles, but maintain the tone and control that is already there.

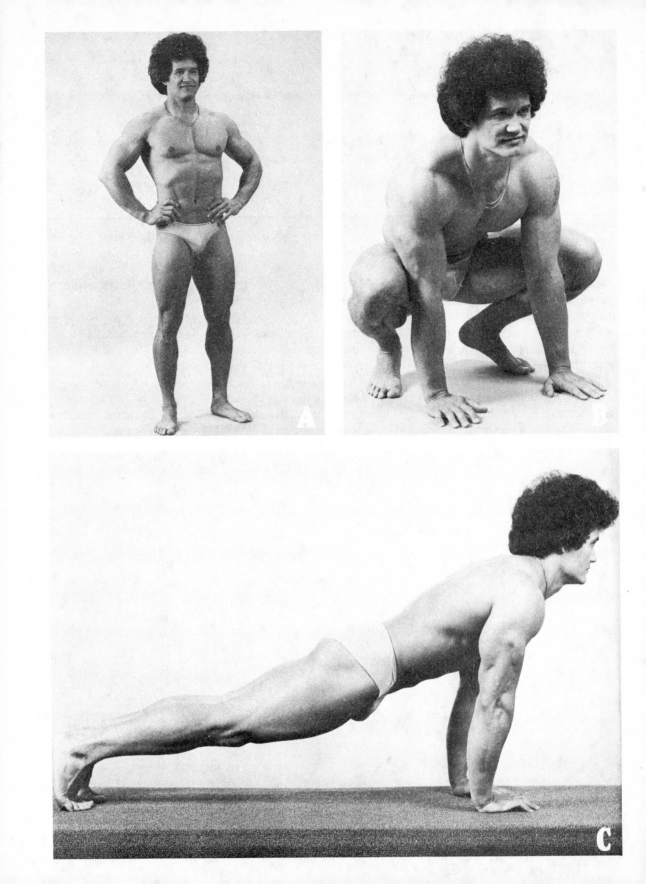

The Frog

A *Starting Position.* Stand with feet apart, hands on hips.

B Lower yourself into a squatting position, arms between the knees, palms on the floor.

C Thrust your legs backward so you land in the push-up position. Reverse the motion so you are back in the squatting position as in **B**.

D Push yourself back up to the starting position and repeat.

Repetitions: 10 (work up to 40).

Benefits: good overall warm-up exercise for all athletes.

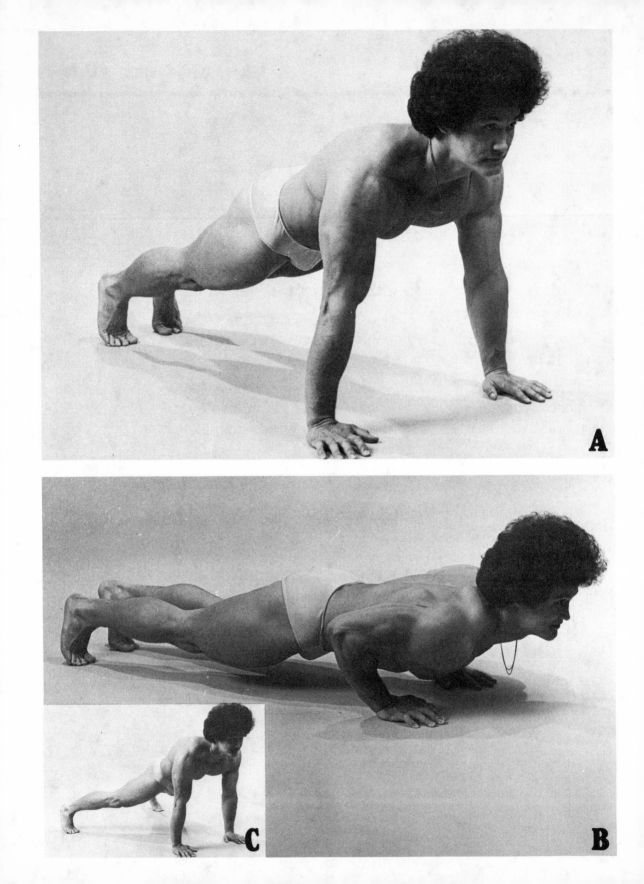

The Hustle

A *Starting Position.* Get into a push-up position, hands wider than shoulder width, feet apart, head up.

B Lower yourself to the floor using the chest and arm muscles. Then push yourself back up. Do two push-ups.

C While in the push-up position, hop your legs open and close twice, then relax and repeat.

Repetitions: 10 (work up to 30).

Benefits: overall conditioning for fast-moving sports.

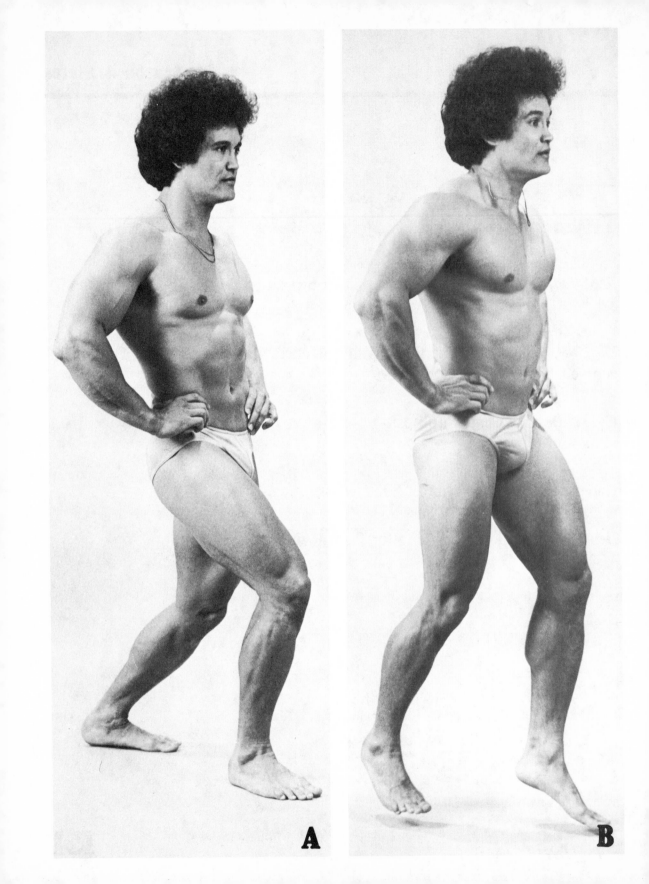

A

B

Lunar Landing

A *Starting Position.* Stand with your knees flexed, one leg ahead of the other, hands on hips, back straight.

B Spring into the air a few inches and land with your leg position reversed.

C Spring again, reverse again, and so on.

Repetitions: 20 (work up to 100).

Benefits: good warm-up exercise and excellent conditioner for leg muscles and respiratory system.

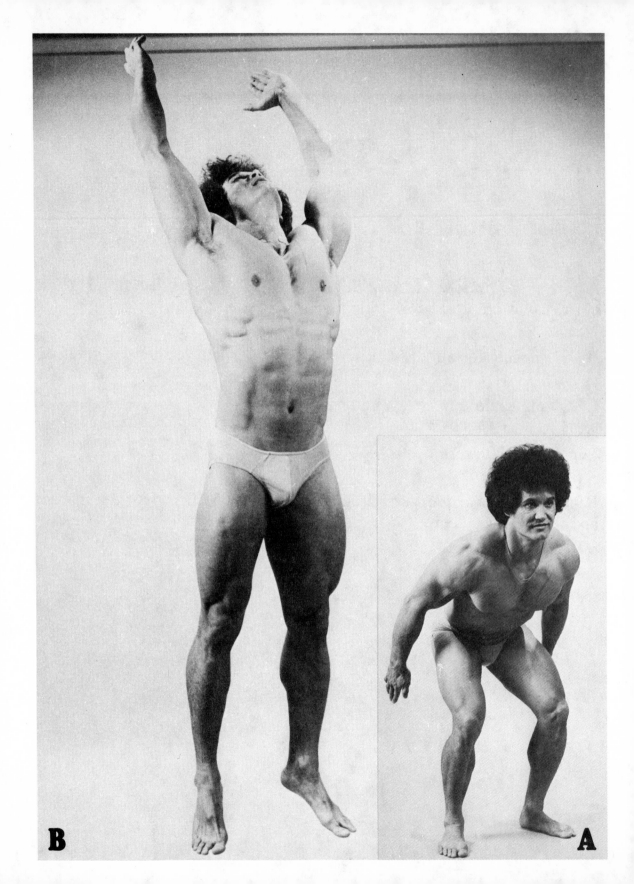

B

A

Picking Apples

A *Starting Position.* Stand with feet apart, knees flexed, bent forward at the waist, hands out and back.

B Leap up as high as you can, swing your arms forward and up, back arched.

C When you land, bring yourself back to the starting position, then spring back up again.

Repetitions: 15 (work up to 40).

Benefits: respiratory system, leg muscles, and shoulder area—overall body stretch.

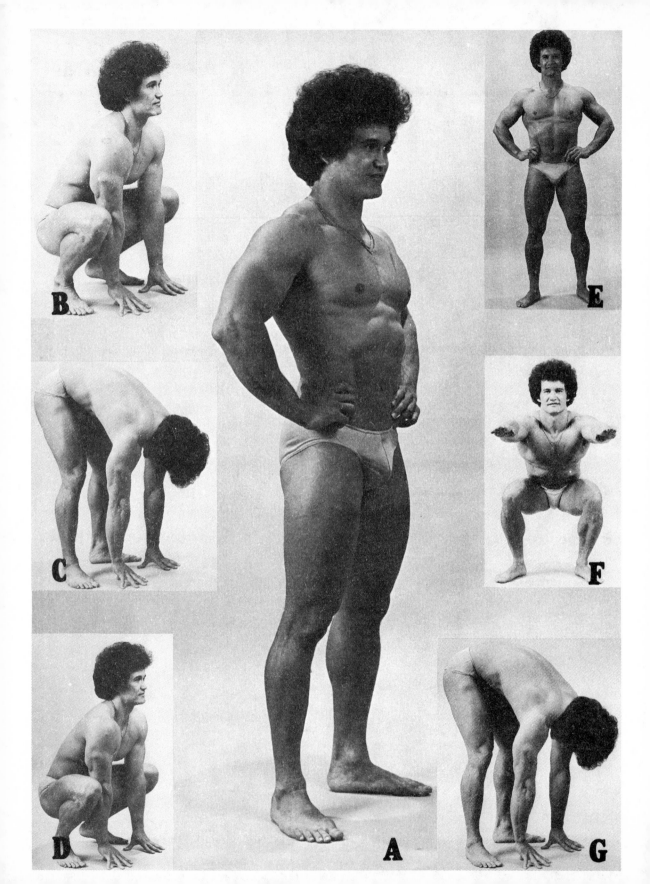

Combination Plate

A *Starting Position.* Stand with your feet spread shoulder width apart, hands on hips.

B Lower yourself into a squatting position, bringing your arms down inside legs, palms on the floor.

C Raise your buttocks up as far as it will go, keeping your fingertips on the floor.

D Return to squatting position.

E Bring yourself back to starting position.

F Lower yourself back to squatting position, swing your arms forward and up (parallel to the floor), palms down. Return to the starting position.

G Bend forward with knees locked, and touch the floor with your fingertips.

H Return to the starting position.

Repetitions: 10 (work up to 30).

Benefits: overall conditioning, especially leg muscles.

157

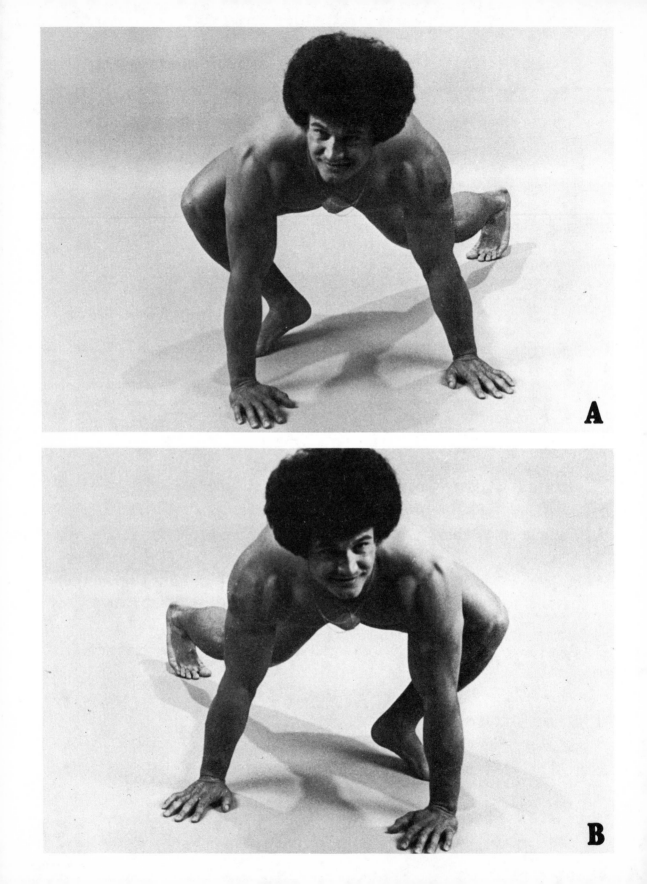

A

B

Running Corkscrew

A *Starting Position.* Get into a modified push-up position, hands shoulder width apart, the right leg forward, and the left leg extended, knee locked. Your legs are at an oblique angle to your body.

B Once you have assumed this position, keep your weight on your hands and alternately thrust your legs out at a forty-five degree angle.

Repetitions: 10 (work up to 50).

Benefits: leg muscles.

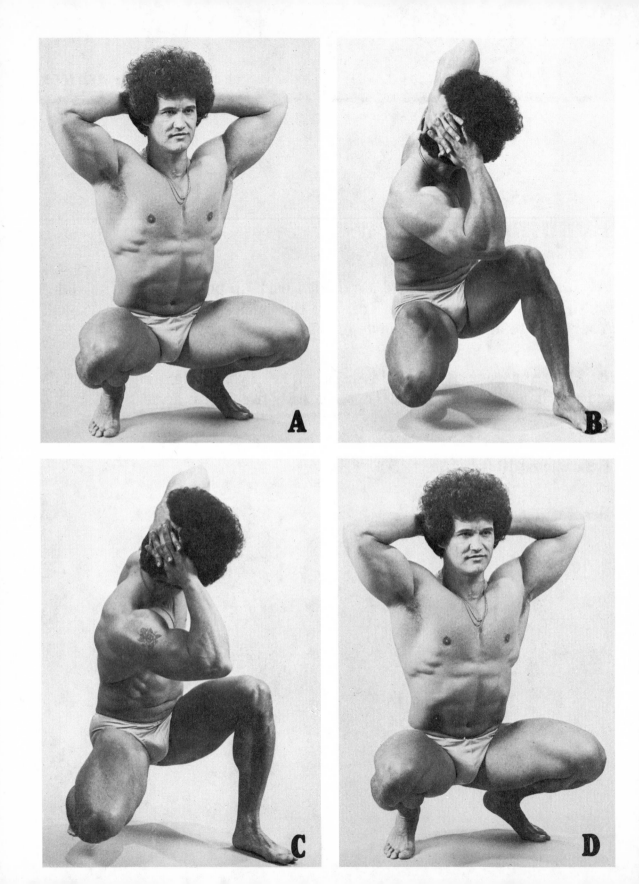

Twisted Duck Walk

A *Starting Position.* Get into a deep squat on your toes, back straight, head up, fingers interlocked behind your head. Staying in the squatting position, walk forward, leading with your right leg. As you move, twist your torso so your left elbow almost touches your right knee.

B Now advance the left leg, twisting your torso toward it, trying to touch your left knee with your right elbow.

Repetitions: 10 (work up to 30).

Benefits: leg and mid-section muscles.

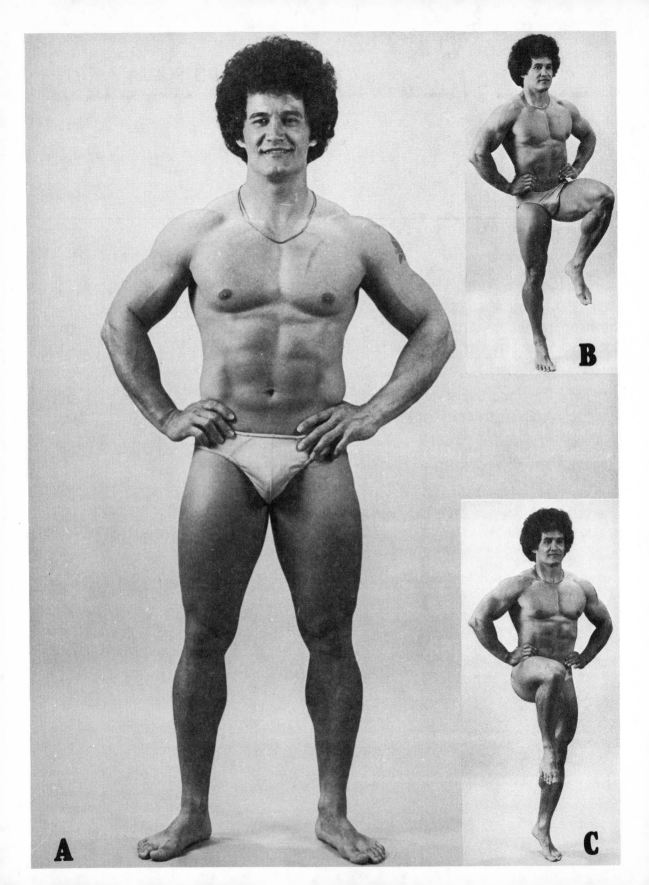

Knee-Highs

A *Starting Position.* Stand with your hands on your hips, feet apart.

B Run in place, but start with a slow pace for about 15 to 20 counts, then raise your knees as far up as you can each time. Push off the floor with a hard hopping motion each time.

Repetitions: 60 (work up to 300).

Benefits: respiratory system, and leg muscles.

PART 3

TRIMMING YOUR PROBLEM AREAS

Parts One and Two of this book contain exercises to tone, tighten, and build up muscle strength. The exercises in this part are designed to help you remove excess fatty tissue from the three most common problem areas—the stomach, buttocks, and waist.

There are seventeen exercises for reducing and flattening the stomach, seven for trimming the waist, and seven to tone and shape the buttocks.

Choose several exercises for your problem area, then add them to your daily routine. Continue to do the extra exercise until your problem is under control.

Remember, however, that all parts of the body must be exercised, toned, and conditioned. When your problem area is under control, you are free to drop the additional exercises, but you must continue your daily routine.

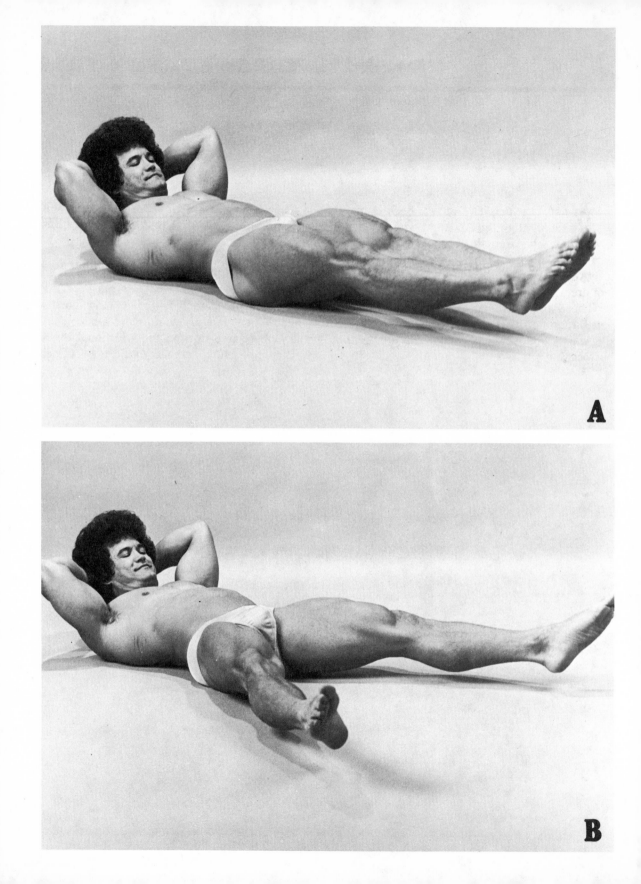

A

B

CHAPTER 8

Stomach Tighteners

Pinchers

A *Starting Position.* Lie on your back on the floor, legs together, hands folded behind your head, fingers interlocked, head up, elbows forward.

B Raise your legs a few inches off the floor and open them as far as possible, toes pointed.

C Pull your legs back to the starting position, keeping your feet off the floor.

Repetitions: 10 (work up to 30).

Also benefits: leg muscles.

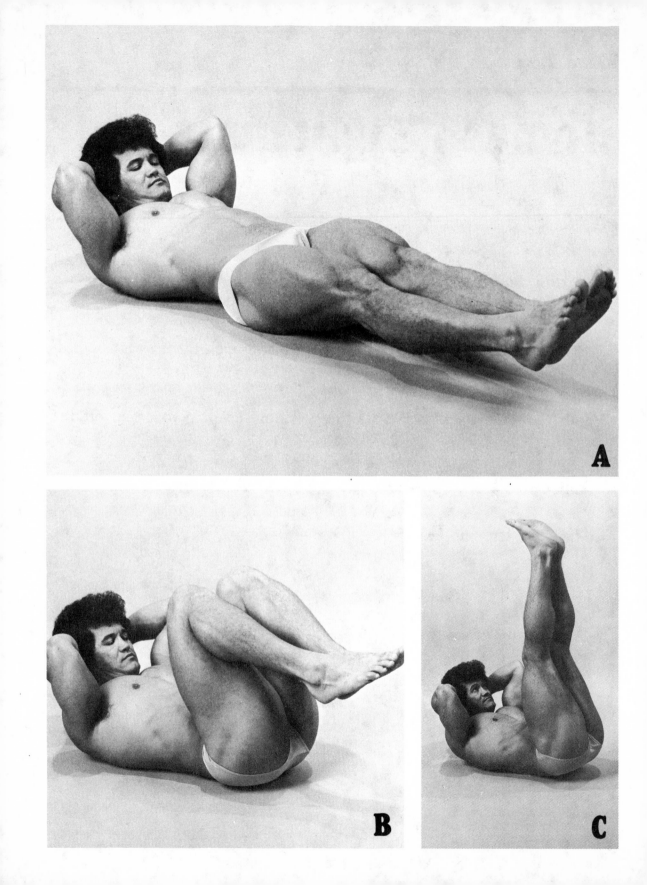

Grasshopper

A *Starting Position.* Lie on the floor, legs extended, knees locked, hands behind your head, fingers interlocked, head up, elbows forward.

B Retract your knees toward your chest as far as possible.

C Bring your legs straight up.

D Lower them to the ground slowly, legs straight, knees locked.

Repetitions: 10 (work up to 20).

Also benefits: leg muscles, buttocks, and stomach.

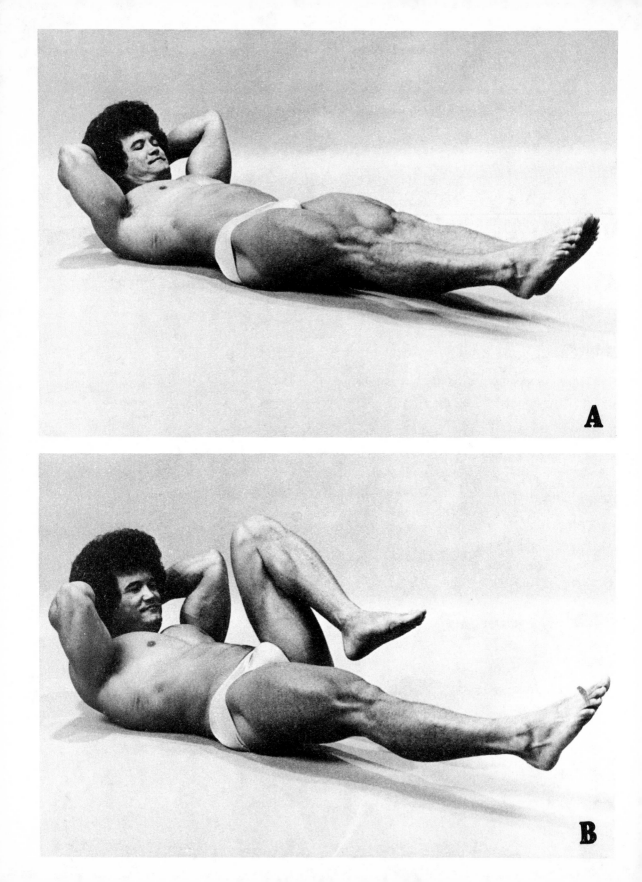

A

B

Bicycle No. 1

A *Starting Position.* Lie on your back, hands behind your head, fingers interlocked, head off the floor.

B Raise your legs off the floor and spin like you are pedaling a bicycle. Extend one leg forward as far as possible, without locking the knee, the knee of the other leg drawn back toward the chest.

Repetitions: 10 (work up to 30).

Also benefits: leg muscle and buttocks.

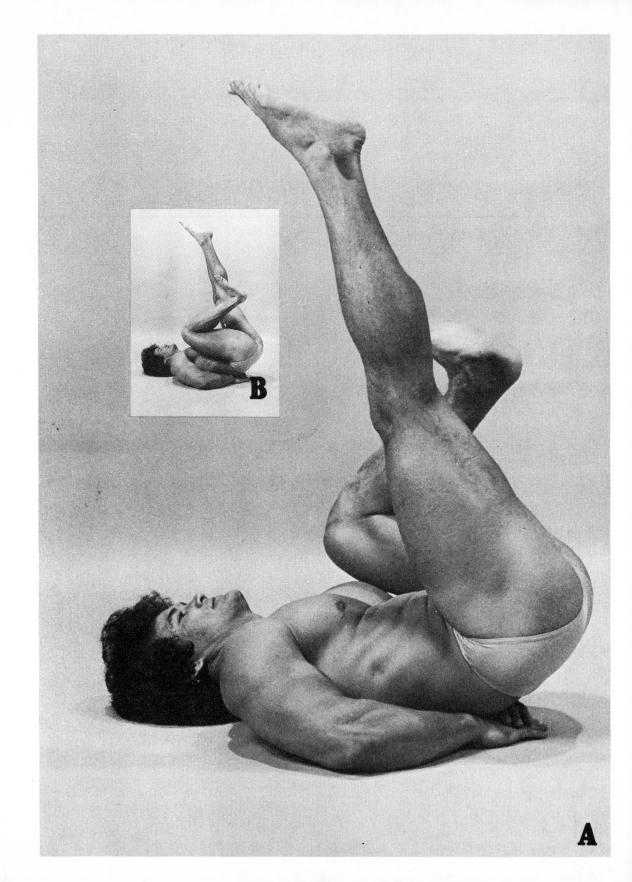

Bicycle No. 2

A *Starting Position.* Lie on your back on the floor, legs together straight up into the air, knees locked, toes pointed. Place your hands under the small of your back for balance. Keep the right leg extended and draw the left leg down toward your chest.

B Make a cycling motion by drawing the right leg down as you straighten the left leg back up.

C Exchange legs in the cycling motion.

Repetitions: 10 (work up to 30).

Also benefits: legs and buttocks.

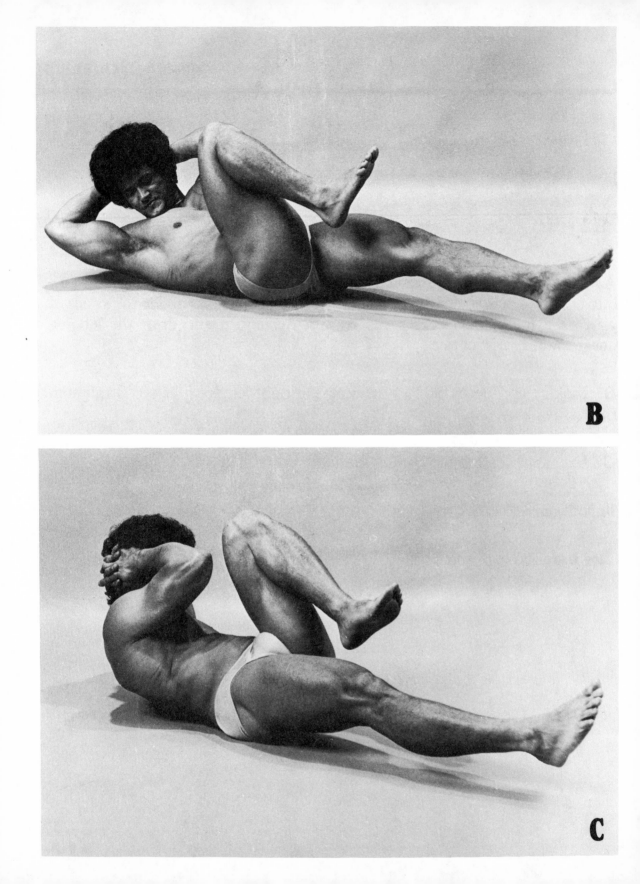

B

C

Steam Engine

A *Starting Position.* Lie on your back, legs together, hands behind your head, fingers interlocked, elbows forward.

B Pull alternate knees up toward your chest, trying to touch them with the opposite elbows.

C The extended leg should be out as far as possible, the knee of the other leg drawn back toward the chest as far as possible.

Repetitions: 10 (work up to 20).

Also benefits: legs, neck, and back muscles.

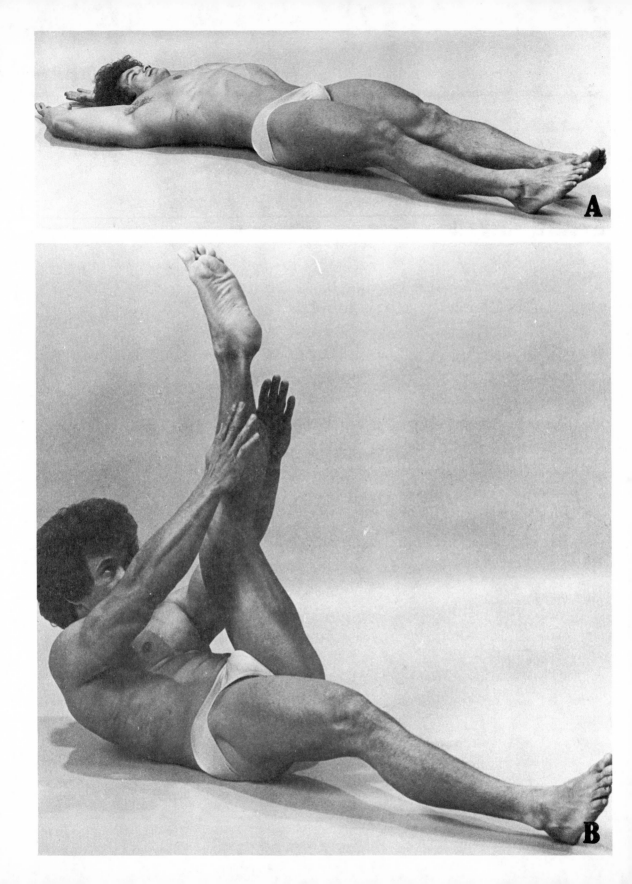

A

B

Cry Baby

A *Starting Position.* Lie on your back, feet together, hands straight up over head.

B Bring the right leg (knees straight or with a slight bend) up as far as possible. At the same time, bring your arms, head, and shoulders off the floor, and attempt to touch your ankles.

C Return to the starting position.

D Repeat the movement with the left leg.

Repetitions: 8 (work up to 15).

Also benefits: back, chest, and legs.

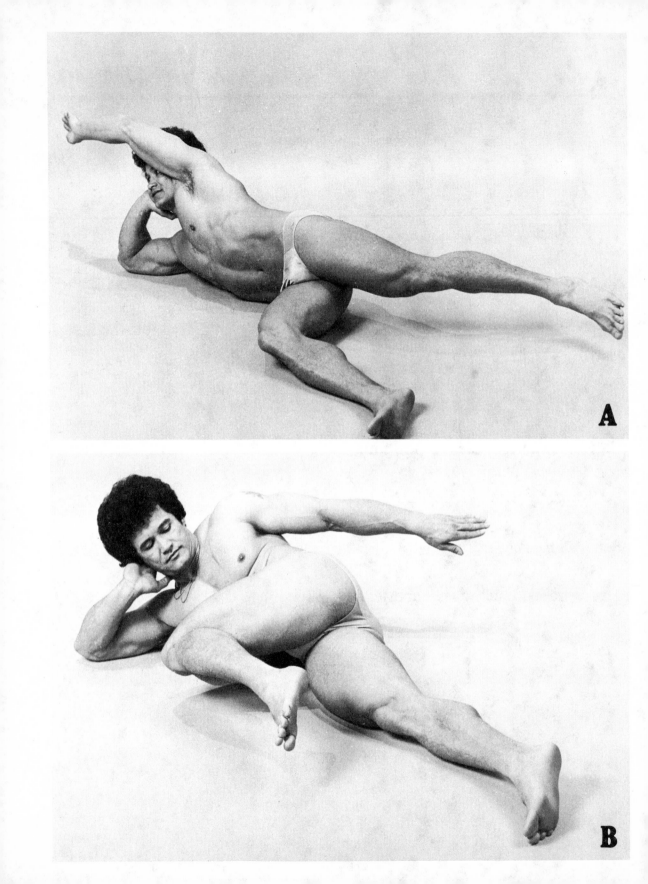

A

B

Express Yourself

A *Starting Position.* Lie on your right side, supporting your head on your right hand, the right leg slightly bent at the knee for balance, the left arm straight up over head, the left leg straight out and pulled back off the floor.

B Swing your left arm forward and to the rear parallel to the floor as you bring your left leg forward, knee bent, toward the chest as far as possible.

C Return to the starting position.

Repetitions: 15 on each side.

Also benefits: chest, shoulders, and back muscles.

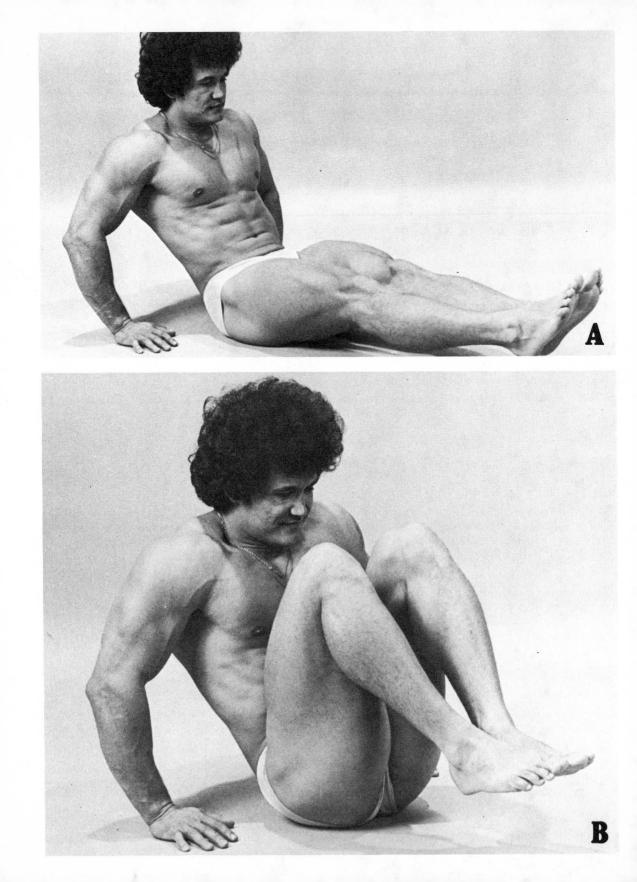

The Bull

A *Starting Position.* Sit on the floor, legs straight out and together, palms on the floor behind your buttocks for balance.

B Raise your legs slightly off the floor and bring your knees up to your chest as far as possible. Return to the starting position, without touching the floor.

Repetitions: 10 (work up to 30).

Also benefits: arms and leg muscles.

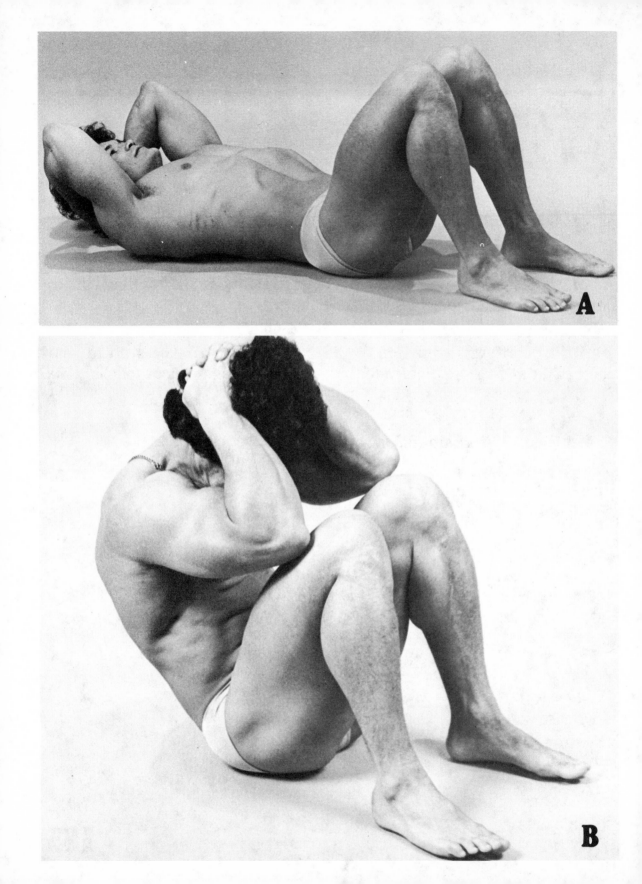

A

B

The Crunch

A *Starting Position.* Lie on the floor with your knees up, hands behind your head, fingers interlocked, elbows forward.

B Pull your torso up, elbows in, trying to touch your head or elbows to your knees.

C Return to the starting position.

Repetitions: 10 (work up to 20).

Also benefits: upper and lower stomach muscles.

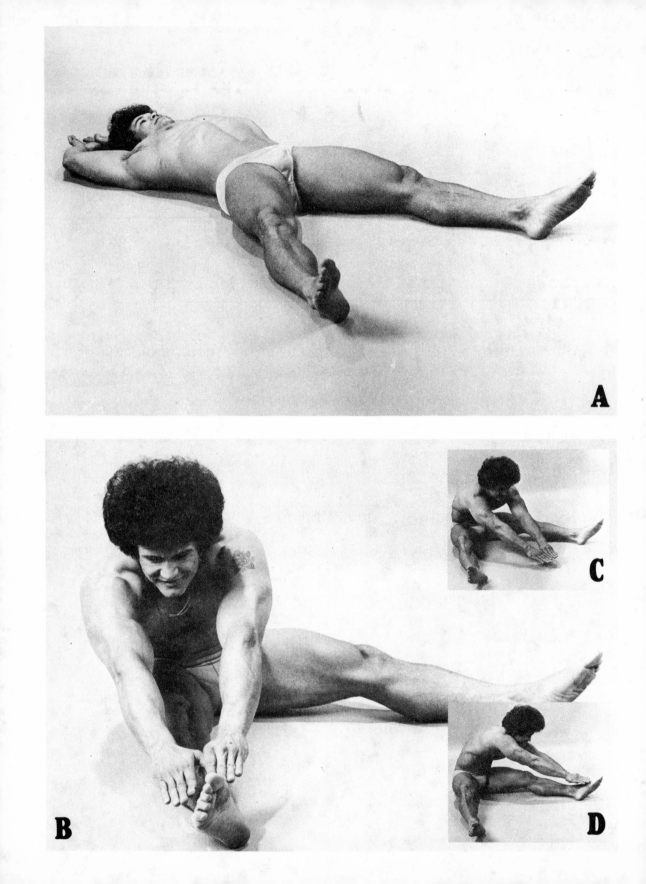

A

B

C

D

Butterfly

A *Starting Position.* Lie on the floor with your legs spread, arms straight out over your head.

B Bring yourself up with elbows locked to the right touching your right toe with your fingertips.

C Swing yourself to the left with a slight bounce touching the floor between your legs, arms straight.

D Take another swing touching your left toe with your fingertips.

E Lower your upper body back to the starting position.

Repetitions: 6 (work up to 12).

Also benefits: back of legs and back muscles.

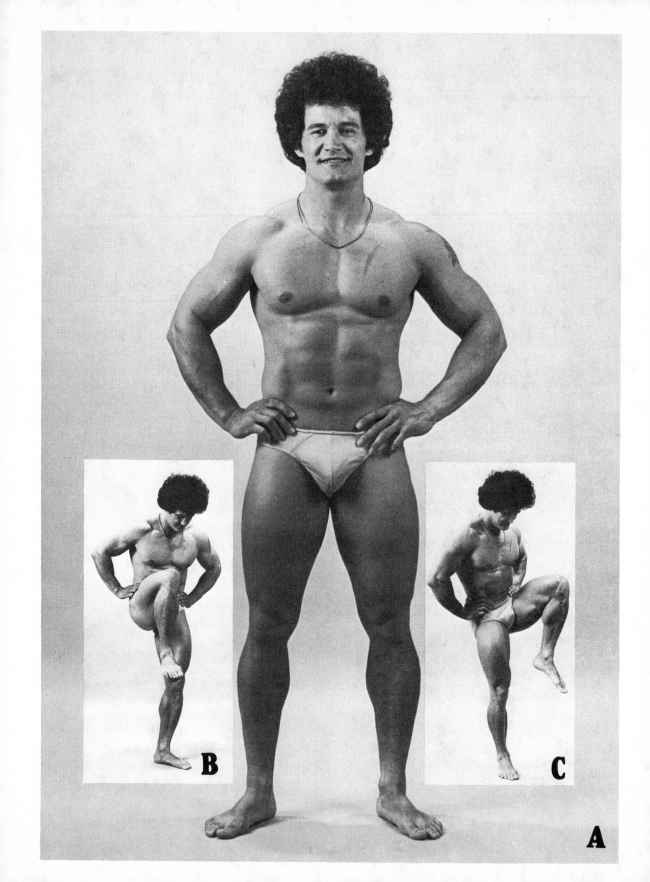

B

C

A

High-Stepper

A *Starting Position.* Stand with your feet spread to shoulder width with hands on your hips.

B Raise one knee as high as possible toward your chest. Hunch forward slightly.

C Alternate legs.

Repetitions: 10 (work up to 30 each leg).

Also benefits: leg muscles.

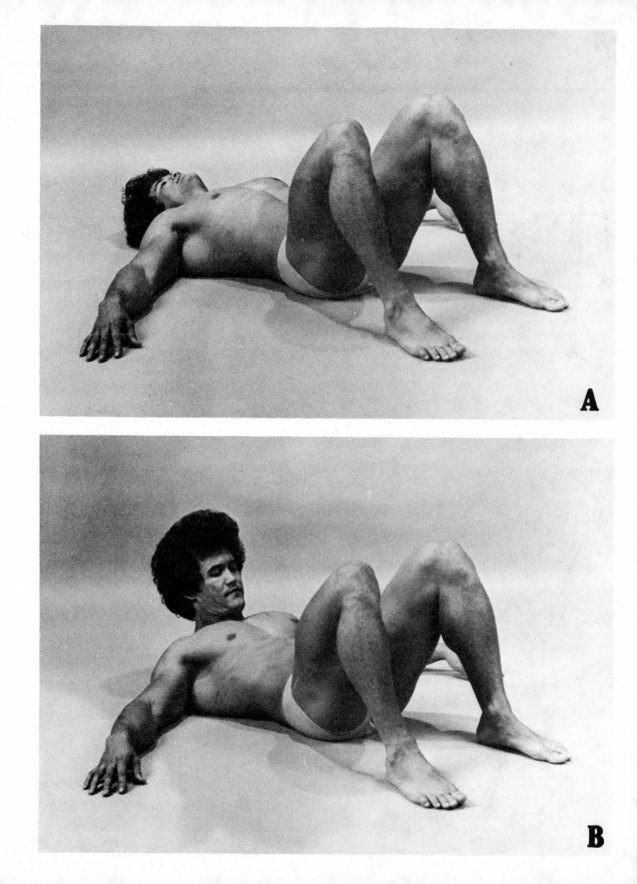

The Hax

A *Starting Position.* Lie on your back, knees bent up and arms to the side.

B Keep the small of your back as flat on the floor as possible, raise your head and tuck your chin in toward your chest.

C Lower your head back to the starting position.

Repetitions: 15 (work up to 30).

Also benefits: upper stomach muscles and chin.

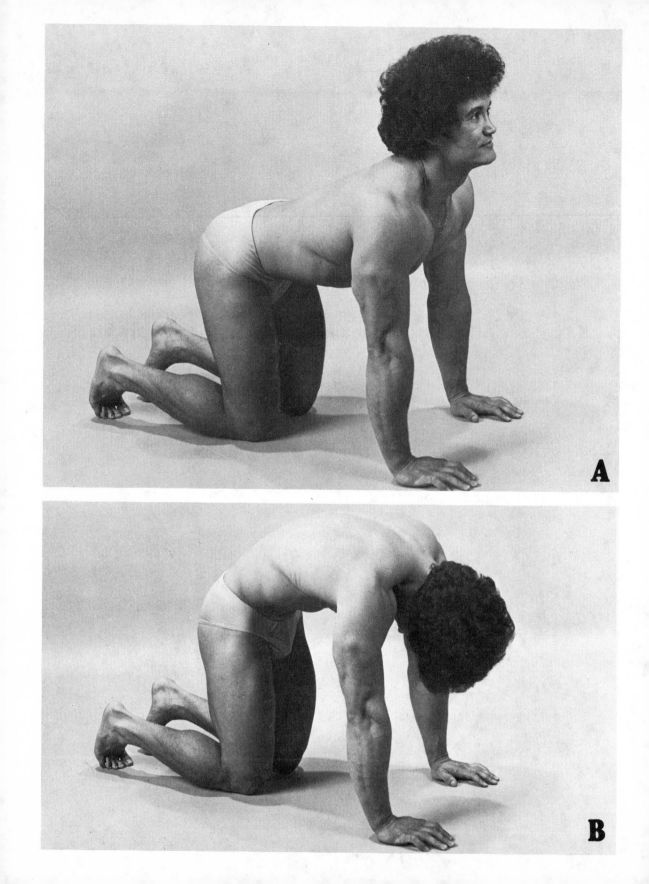

A

B

Buckeroo

A *Starting Position.* Get down on your hands and knees with your head up.

B Tuck your head between your arms and arch your back, contracting the stomach muscles at the same time.

C Return to starting position.

Repetitions: 10 (work up to 30).

Also benefits: back and neck muscles.

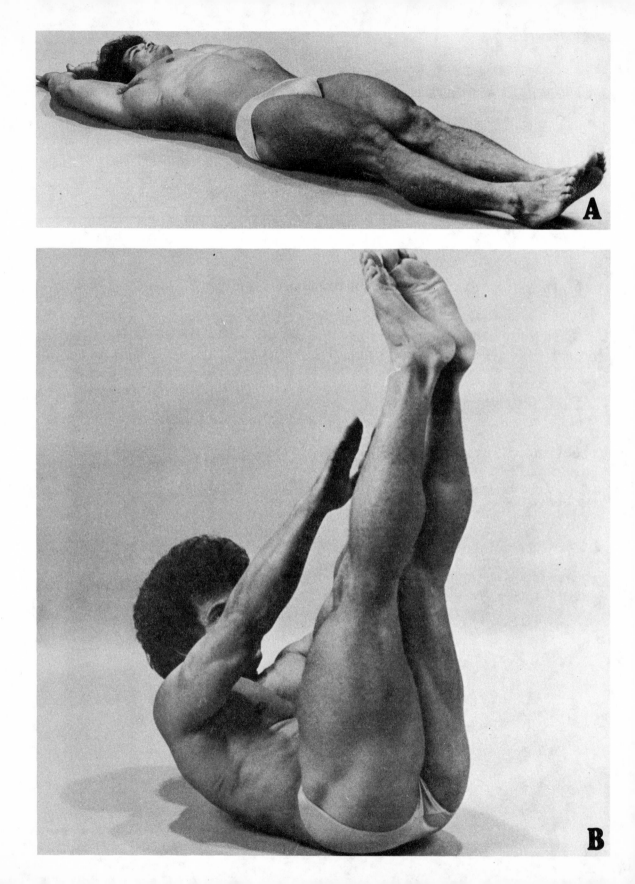

The Dive

A *Starting Position.* Lie on the floor with your arms over your head, thumbs locked, legs together, and knees locked.

B Raise your arms and legs and attempt to touch your ankles.

C Lower yourself to the starting position.

Repetitions: 6 (work up to 12).

Also benefits: chest, leg, and back muscles.

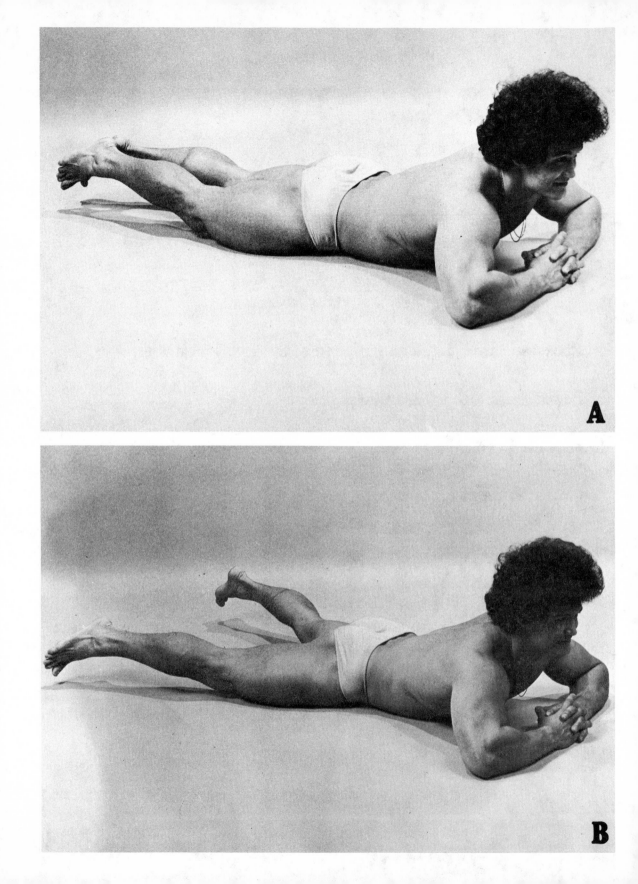

A

B

CHAPTER 9

Buttocks Shapers

The Swimmer

A *Starting Position.* Lie on your stomach, arms folded under chin, fingers interlocked. Raise your legs off the floor with your knees locked.

B Open your legs as far as possible.

C Close your legs strongly, touching your heels on the closing motion.

Repetitions: 10 (work up to 50).

Also benefits: lower back, leg, and stomach muscles.

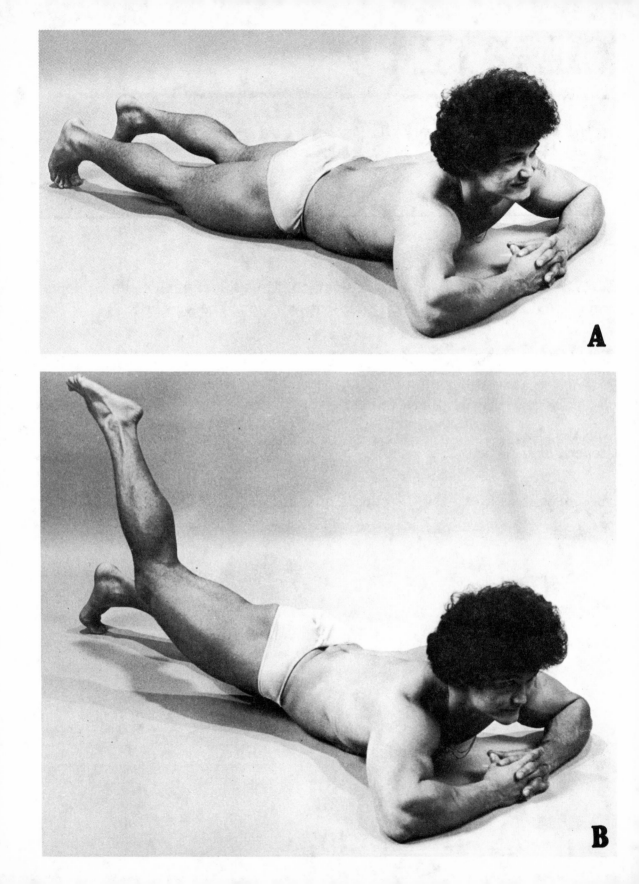

A

B

Leg Lifts

A *Starting Position.* Lie on your stomach, arms folded under chin, fingers interlocked. Knees should be slightly bent or locked.

B Raise the right leg up high.

C Return to the starting position, and repeat with left leg.

Repetitions: 15 (work up to 30 each leg).

Also benefits: lower back and leg muscles.

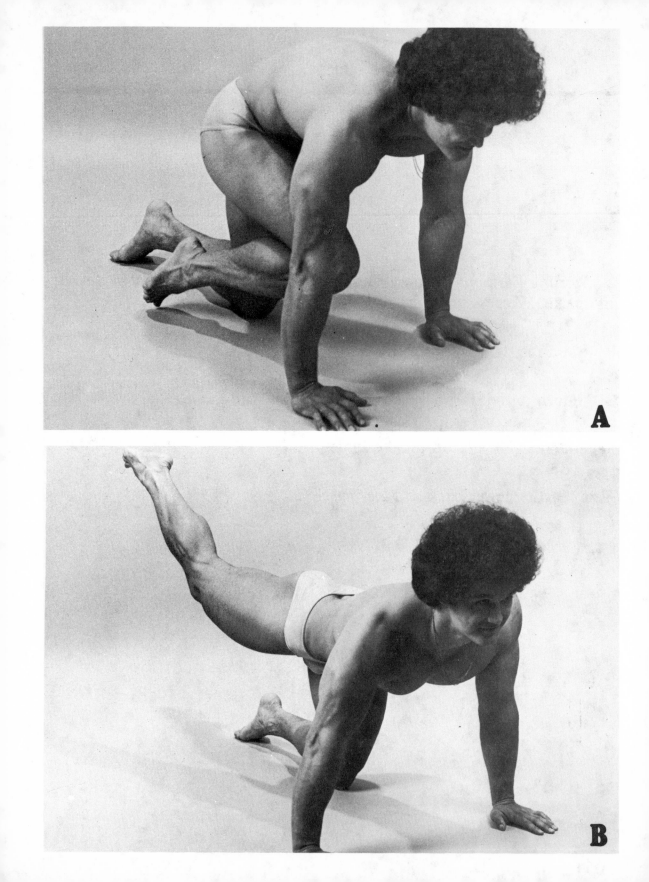

A

B

Cam Shaft

A *Starting Position.* Get down on your hands and knees, the right knee off the floor and under your chest, head up, and hands shoulder width apart.

B Kick the right leg straight back and upward.

C Return to the starting position and repeat.

Repetitions: 20 (work up to 40).

Also benefits: stomach and back muscles.

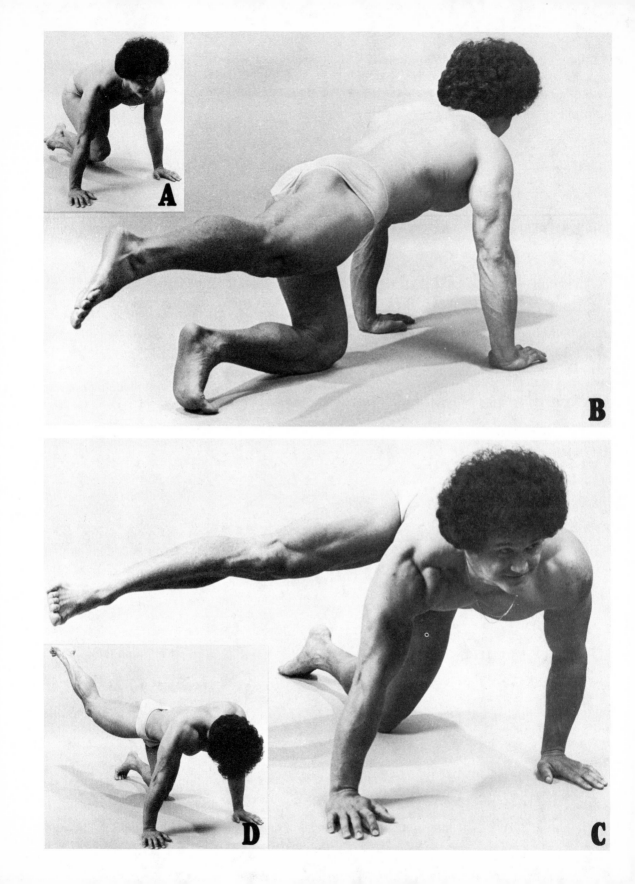

Side-Kicker

A *Starting Position.* Get down on your hands and knees, the right knee off the floor and under the chest, head up, and hands shoulder width apart.

B Kick straight back with the right leg.

C Rotate your hip and leg outward and around so that it is at a ninety degree angle to your body, eyes on your toes.

D Bring the leg back to the extended position. Then return to starting position.

Repetitions: 10 (work up to 20).

Also benefits: waist, leg, stomach, and back muscles.

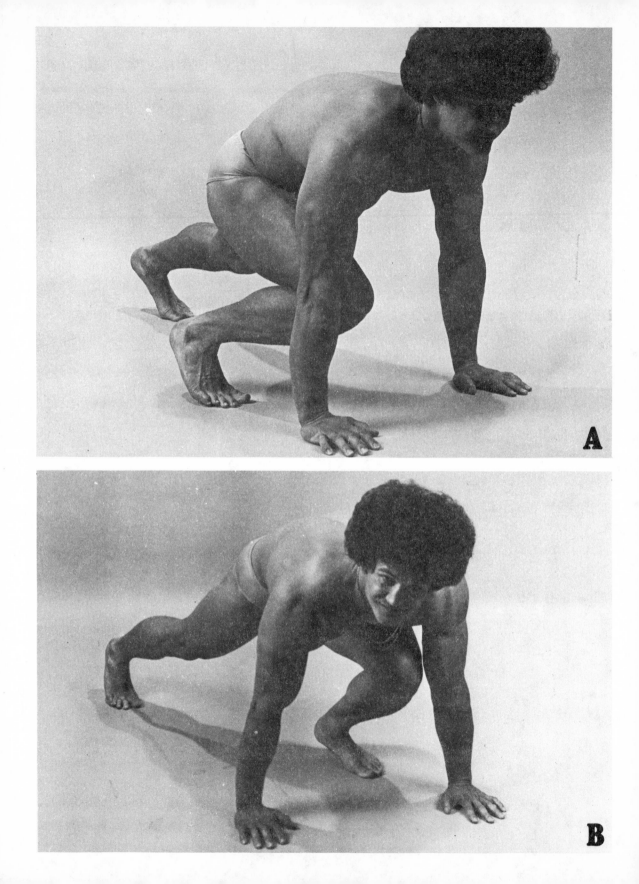

A

B

Mountain Climber

A *Starting Position.* Position yourself as though you were about to take off in a sprint. Hands should be flat on the floor, the right knee on the inside of the right elbow, the left leg extended straight back, head up.

B Reverse the position of the legs. Try to keep your buttocks from bouncing up high into the air.

Repetitions: 20 (work up to 50).

Also benefits: stomach, arms, and back muscles.

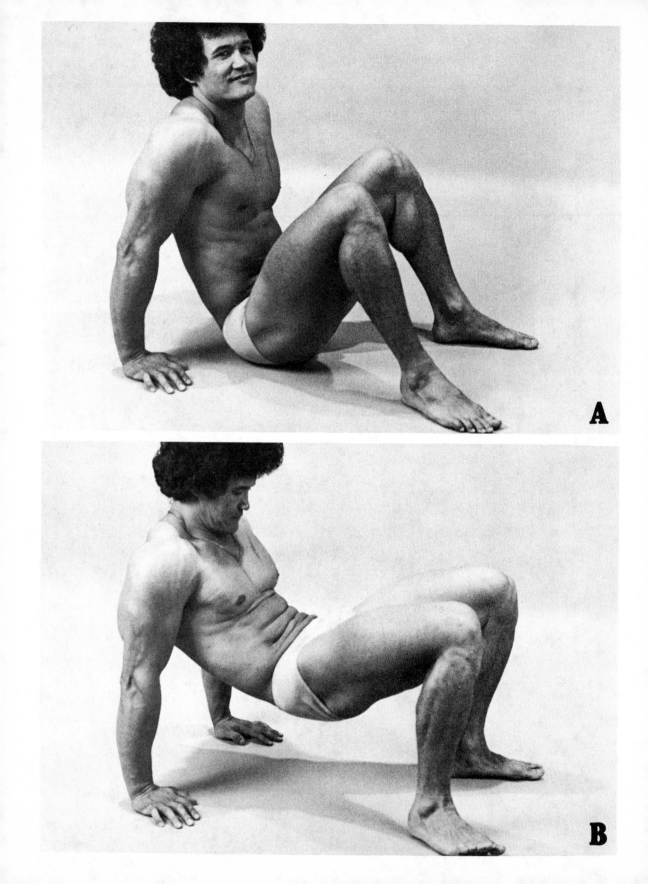

A

B

Risers

A *Starting Position.* Sit on the floor with your legs spread, knees drawn up, hands behind your hips, palms flat, fingers pointing to the front for balance.

B Raise yourself up as far as possible. Tighten the buttocks muscles.

C Return to the starting position, relax, and rise up again.

Repetitions: 10 (work up to 20).

Also benefits: back of the arms, back, stomach, and lower leg muscles.

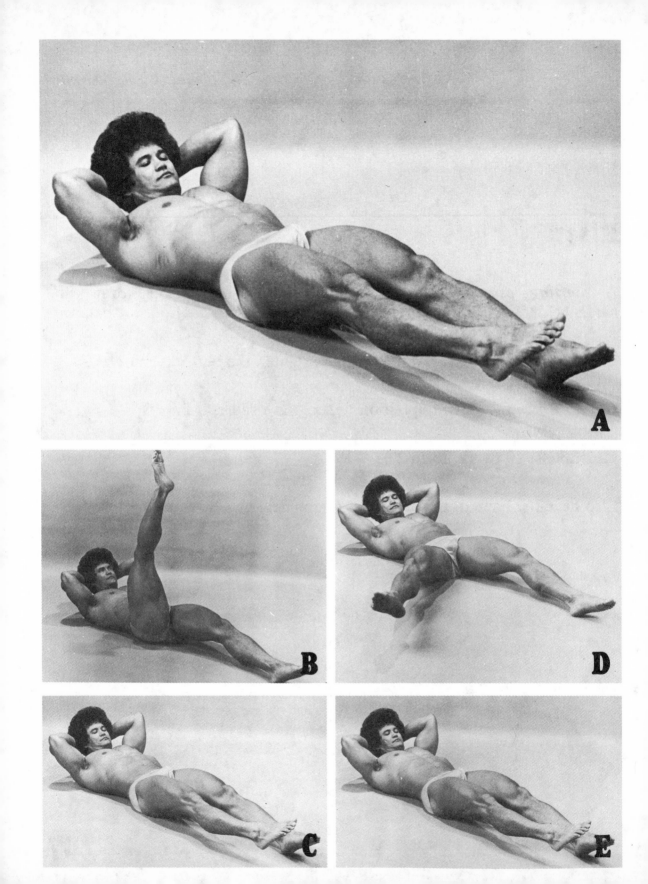

Half Scissors

A *Starting Position.* Lie on your back on the floor, hands behind your neck, head up, fingers interlocked.

B Raise the right leg straight up. Knees should be straight or slightly bent.

C Lower the leg to the starting position, without touching the floor.

D Kick the right leg out to the side as far as possible. Try to keep your back flat on the floor.

E Return to the starting position.

Repetitions: 10 (work up to 20).

Also benefits: leg and stomach muscles.

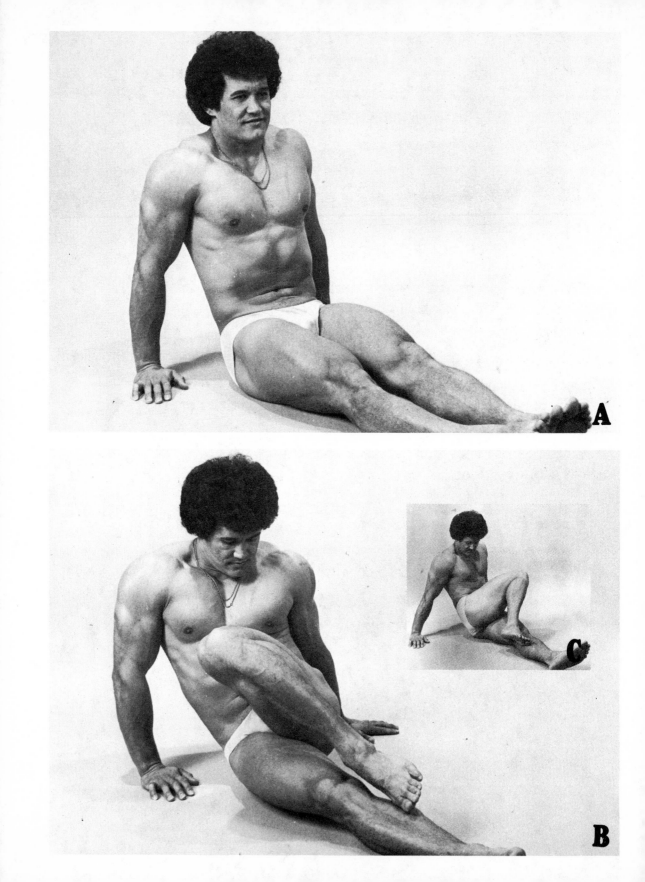

A

B

C

CHAPTER 10

Waist Trimmers

Rock the Boat

A *Starting Position.* Sit on the floor, legs extended, hands behind your buttocks, palms on the floor for balance.

B Keeping your legs together, rotate over on your left thigh, at the same time bringing your right knee up toward your chest by sliding your right foot up over the left leg. Return to the starting position.

C Rotate to the right side, and repeat exercise.

D Return to the starting position.

Repetitions: 6 (work up to 20).

Also benefits: stomach muscles.

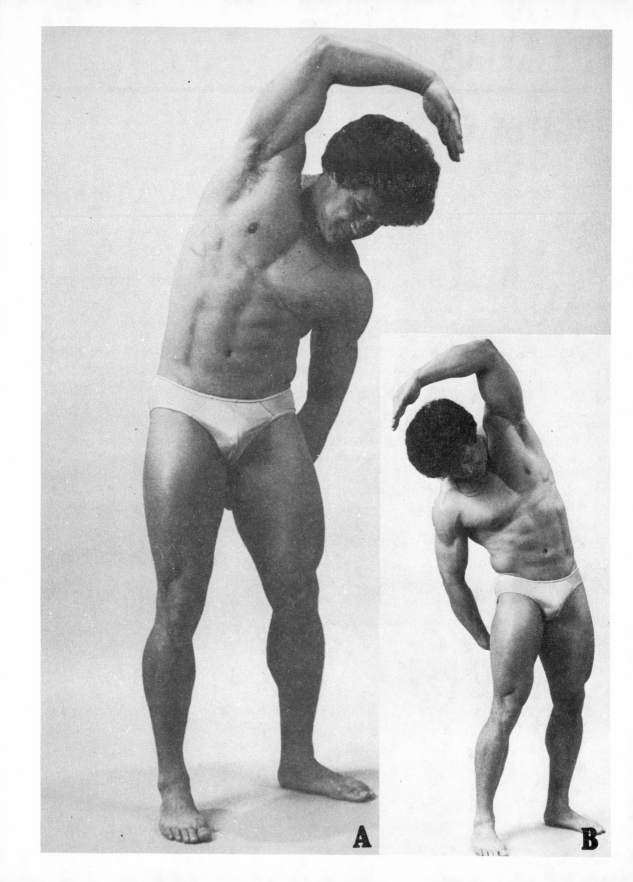

A

B

Broken Windmill

A *Starting Position.* Stand with your feet apart to shoulder width, the right arm up over your head, hand cupped, slight bend at the elbow, the left arm is down behind your buttocks.

B Swing side-to-side in a circular motion.

Repetitions: 10 (work up to 30).

Also benefits: upper back muscles and stomach muscles.

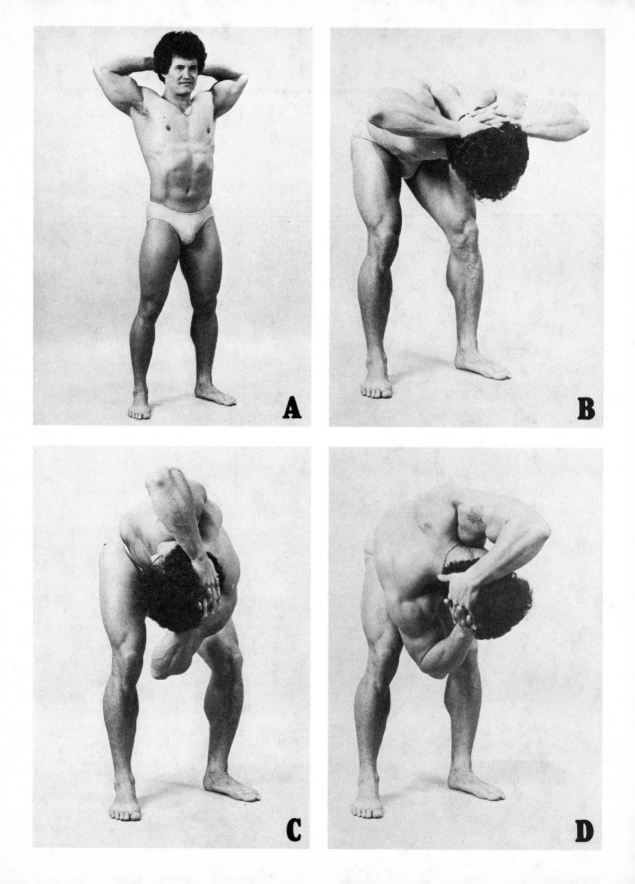

Pit-Bull

A *Starting Position.* Stand with your feet apart, hands behind your neck, fingers interlocked, knees slightly bent, and elbows back.

B Bend forward at the waist, elbows stay back, back straight.

C Twist strongly to the left side, attempting to touch your left knee with the right elbow.

D Twist strongly to the right side.

E Return to the starting position.

Repetitions: 10 (work up to 30).

Also benefits: back of legs, lower back, and stomach muscles.

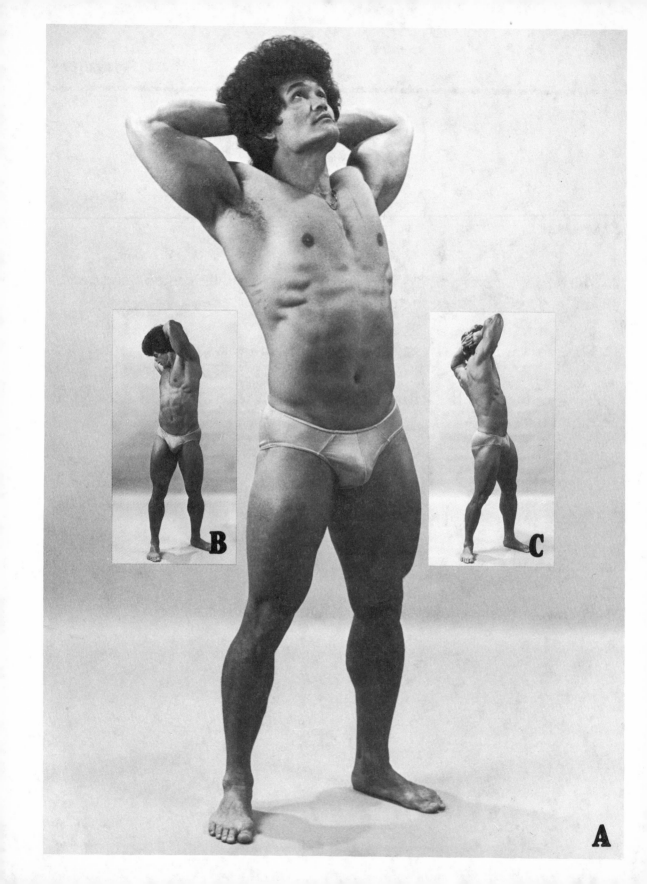

B

C

A

Backward Twist

A *Starting Position.* Stand with your legs spread to shoulder width, your fingers interlocked behind your head. With elbows out, arch your back and look up.

B Twist strongly to the right, looking at your right heel as you turn.

C Twist strongly to the other side.

Repetitions: 10 (work up to 20).

Also benefits: back and stomach muscles.

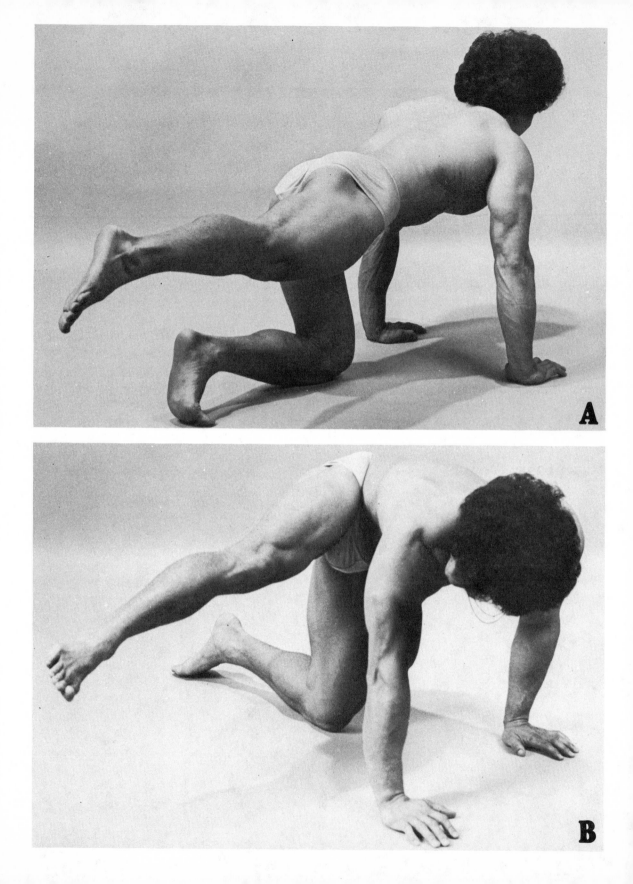

A

B

The Tail Wag

A *Starting Position.* Get on your hands and knees, extend your right leg straight back parallel with the floor, knee locked.

B Swing your leg to the right at about a ninety degree angle to your body and look at your right toe.

C Swing your right leg back over to the left side and look at your left toe.

Repetitions: 10 (work up to 20).

Also benefits: neck, lower back muscles, and buttocks.

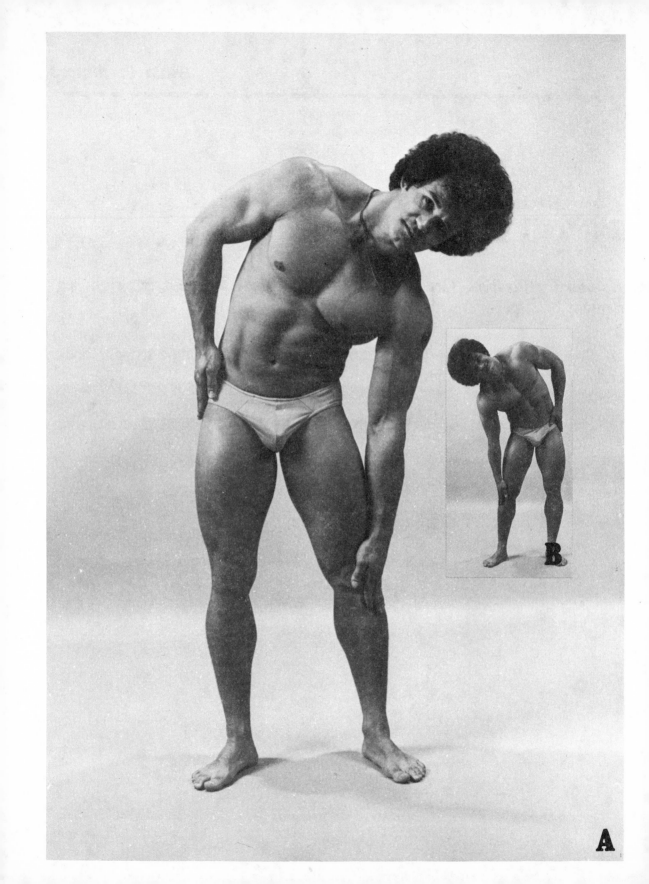

A

Saturday Night Fever

A *Starting Position.* Stand with your legs spread to shoulder width, palms against your thighs. Bend slightly forward. (Bending forward or backward, or standing straight changes the muscle doing the work.)

B Bend to the right side, running your hands up and down your thighs as far as possible.

C Bend to the left side.

Repetitions: 20 (work up to 40).

Also benefits: stomach muscles.

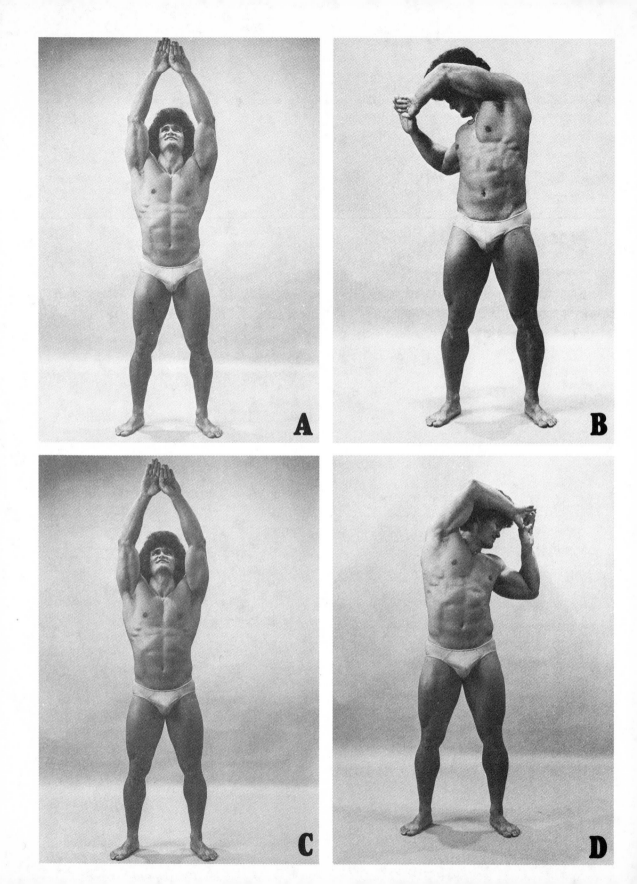

The Row Boat

A *Starting Position.* Stand with your legs spread to shoulder width, head up, arms straight over the head, and thumbs locked together.

B Twist your upper body to the right, pulling your right elbow down as far as possible, turning your head and looking at the floor between your arms and body.

C Return to the starting position.

D Twist your upper body to the left.

E Return to the starting position.

Repetitions: 10 (work up to 20).

Also benefits: back muscle and chest.

Recommended Reading

Davis, Adelle. *Let's Eat Right to Keep Fit.* New York: New American Library, 1970.

Editors of *Runner's World. New Exercises for Runners.* Mountain View, Calif.: World Publications, 1978.

Editors of *Runner's World. The Runner's Diet.* Rev. ed. Mountain View, Calif.: World Publications, 1978.

Fleck, Henrietta. *Introduction to Nutrition.* 2nd edition. New York: Macmillan Publishing Co., Inc., 1976.

Higdon, Hal, ed. *Complete Diet Guide for Runners and Other Athletes.* Mountain View, Calif.: World Publications, 1978.

Higdon, Hal. *Beginner's Running Guide.* Mountain View, Calif.: World Publications, 1978.

Kirschmann, John D. *Nutrition Almanac.* New York: McGraw-Hill Book Co., 1975.

LaLanne, Jack. *Foods for Glamour.* New York: Arc Books, 1970.

Miller, Marjorie. *Introduction to Health Food.* New York: Dell Publishing Co., Inc., 1972.

Null, Gary, et al. *The Complete Question and Answer Book of General Nutrition.* 2nd edition. New York: Dell Publishing Co., Inc., 1974.

Robinson, Corinne H. *Fundamentals of Normal Nutrition.* 2nd edition. Edited by Joan C. Zulch. New York: Macmillan Publishing Co., Inc., 1973.

Williams, Sue Rodwell. *Nutrition and Diet Therapy.* 2nd edition. St. Louis: C. V. Mosby Company, 1973.

About the Author

Benny Crawford has been interested in recreational exercise since childhood days in his native Guam. Following a disabling back injury that ended his military career, Crawford concentrated on body building and exercise as a form of rehabilitation. In 1976 he won the Mr. California title at the International Federation of Body Building championships.

His other activities include sky diving, bicycling, running, table tennis, and racquetball.

Crawford currently resides with his wife, Kathryn, and their two children, Elisha and Zion, in San Leandro, California, where he is president of the New World Gym. He is also a recreation major at San Francisco State University.

The *Book for Every Body* is his first book.